Nanomedicinal Approaches Towards Cardiovascular Disease

Edited by

Fahima Dilnawaz
Laboratory of Nanomedicine
Institute of Life Sciences
Bhubaneswar, Odisha, India

&

Zeenat Iqbal
Department of Pharmaceutics
School of Pharmaceutical Education and Research
Jamia Hamdard, New Delhi, India

Nanomedicinal Approaches Towards Cardiovascular Disease

Editors: Fahima Dilnawaz and Zeenat Iqbal

ISBN (Online): 978-981-4998-21-5

ISBN (Print): 978-981-4998-22-2

ISBN (Paperback): 978-981-4998-23-9

need for a court order if at any point you breach any terms of this License Agreement. In no event will any delay or failure by Bentham Science Publishers in enforcing your compliance with this License Agreement constitute a waiver of any of its rights.

3. You acknowledge that you have read this License Agreement, and agree to be bound by its terms and conditions. To the extent that any other terms and conditions presented on any website of Bentham Science Publishers conflict with, or are inconsistent with, the terms and conditions set out in this License Agreement, you acknowledge that the terms and conditions set out in this License Agreement shall prevail.

Bentham Science Publishers Pte. Ltd.
80 Robinson Road #02-00
Singapore 068898
Singapore
Email: subscriptions@benthamscience.net

**BENTHAM
SCIENCE**

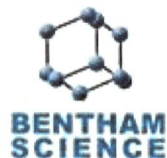

CONTENTS

FOREWORD 1

It is my immense pleasure to write the foreword to this book. The book deals with various aspects of nanotechnology based application for the treatment of cardiovascular disease.

Across the globe cardiac diseases remain the major cause of mortality and morbidity despite current pharmacological advancements, however, a complete cure for the disease has not been accomplished. In cardiac therapy nanotechnology-based therapeutic application has illustrated remarkable progress. Immense usefulness of nanotechnological application towards therapy, it is highly anticipated that nanomedicine may fill the huge gap by initializing the new avenues to meet the existing therapeutic demands of cardiovascular diseases. And it may provide a subtle solution with better prognoses along with a reduced side effect profile.

This abreast book is quite informative as it deals with the understanding of the cardiovascular disease and current progression of nanotechnological mode for the holistic approach of the therapeutic improvement. This book gives the surfeit information about various nanocarriers, biomaterials for cardiac tissue regeneration which is highly beneficial for the students, academicians and clinicians. The simple language with pictorial illustration of the book will surely help for the upgraded understanding of the subject.

I am convinced that my colleagues *Dr. Fahima Dilnawaz* and *Dr. Zeenat Iqbal* have done a great, focused and detailed job in compiling and editing this cutting edge and comprehensive book on nanomedicine and cardiovascular disorders written by subject experts. I wish this extraordinary book to entice extensive readership, and I hope the readers will thoroughly enjoy the assortment of recent scientific facts as much as I did!

Farida Khan
Department of Biochemistry
Sir Seewoosagur Ramgoolam Medical College
Mauritius

FOREWORD 2

It is a pleasure to write the foreword to this book. It presents a comprehensive review of various aspects of nanotechnology in the treatment, drug delivery and amelioration of cardiovascular disease.

Up till now, cardiac diseases remain the major cause of mortality and morbidity across the globe and despite the recent therapeutics' options and pharmacological advancements, a complete cure for cardiac diseases has not yet been achieved. However, in recent years, a tremendous explosion has been seen in the advancement of nanotechnology, where nanomedicine has brought a remarkable improvement in cardiac therapy. And it is expected that nanomedicine will fill the remaining gap by opening new frontiers for inventing newer therapies and addressing the unmet needs of cardiovascular diseases.

This up-to-date book incorporates both the underlying science of cardiovascular diseases and the advancements in the field of nanotechnology in such a balanced fashion that led to the holistic development in the next generation of disease treatment. From nanocarriers to biomaterials for cardiac tissue regeneration, this book gives a plethora of information that will be definitely beneficial for the students and clinicians. Also, simple language and pictorial presentations of the various concepts will help in the better dissemination of knowledge and hence a better understanding of the book.

I am convinced that *Dr. Fahima Dilnawaz* and *Dr. Zeenat Iqbal* have done a great, focused and detailed job in compiling and editing this cutting edge and comprehensive book on nanomedicine and cardiovascular disorders, written by subject matter experts from academia. I wish this extraordinary book attracts a broad readership and I hope the readers will enjoy this collection of scientific facts as much as I did.

Shamarez Ali Mohammed
Dr. Reddy's Laboratories
India

PREFACE

The last decade has witnessed a tremendous change in the way disease therapy has been impacted by nanotechnology. It has indeed birthed and nurtured a newer branch of advanced therapy and diagnostics vis a vis "**nanomedicine**" . The uniqueness and propensity of adapting itself to diagnosis and treatment of plethora of diseases makes "**nanomedicine**" a key area of pharmaceutical research. Although at its nascent stage "**the nanomedicine approaches as an intervention for cardiac diseases**", is fast attracting the attention of researchers and practitioners alike. Cardiac diseases are often associated with myriad complications during the lifetime of a patient and continue to remain the cause of frequent deaths worldwide. The disease segment is still on a lookout of well-equipped treatment tools and is poised to explore nanomedicine armamentarium wherein, cardiovascular complications could be diagnosed at the molecular level and its treatment is delivered at the cellular level. This, precisely would make a fit case for early detection and diagnosis followed by quicker remedy for the cardiac ailments. This would indeed be a welcome step as most cardiac diseases often reduce the window of survival time for the patients.

The book entitled "**Nanomedicinal approaches for cardiovascular disease**" by **Dr. Fahima Dilnawaz and Dr. Zeenat Iqbal** illustrates the application of nanomedicine and nanotechnology in the diagnosis and treatment of cardiovascular diseases. This book indeed is a humble attempt to present the various approaches of nanomedicine in cardiovascular ailments to the broad readership, including academicians, researchers, scholars and clinicians. The authors have made concerted efforts towards inviting various reputed contributors who have been working in the domain of nanomedicine for quite some time.

This book is divided into separate sections such as: Section 1: *Introduction to cardiovascular diseases and need of nanomedicine and regenerative nanomedicine: Nanomedicine aspects in cardiovascular diseases, Role of Nanomedicine in the diagnosis of cardiovascular diseases, Nanotechnology based molecular imaging in cardiovascular disease, Nanocarriers for therapeutics delivery of cardiovascular diseases, Nanocarriers for theranostics delivery of cardiovascular diseases, Nanocarriers for biologicals delivery to cardiovascular delivery and Ethics and regulations for cardiovascular diseases.* Section 2: *Biomaterials for cardiac regeneration, Biomimetic materials design for cardiac tissue regeneration, Nanotechnology based direct cardiac reprogramming for cardiac regeneration, Smart nanomaterials for cardiac regeneration therapy, Stem cell engineering ability to promote cardiac regenerative activity.*

Each section gives a plethora of novel information on a particular field. Summarily, the book is a collection of quality information on various applications of nanomedicine that can be applied for the successful treatment of cardiovascular diseases. The lucid textual and pictorial presentation of the various sections and chapters is primarily in simple language that will support easy dissemination of knowledge.

The authors are hopeful that the collaborative efforts invested in the writing of this book on a very dedicated area of nanomedicine in cardiac diseases would attract good readership.

Fahima Dilnawaz
Department Laboratory of Nanomedicine
Institute of Life Sciences
Bhubaneswar, Odisha
India

&

Zeenat Iqbal
Department of Pharmaceutics
School of Pharmaceutical Education
and Research (SPER)
Jamia Hamdard, New Delhi
India

List of Contributors

Ajit Kumar Behura   Department of Humanities and Social Sciences, Indian Institute of Technology (ISM) Dhandbad, Dhandbad-826004, Jharkhand, India

Fahima Dilnawaz   Laboratory of Nanomedicine, Institute of Life Sciences, Nalco Square, Chandrasekharpur, Bhubaneswar-751023, Odisha, India

Foziyah Zakir   Department of Pharmaceutics, Nanomedicine Laboratory, School of Pharmaceutical Education and Research, Jamia Hamdard, New Delhi-110062, India Department of Pharmaceutics, School of Pharmaceutical Sciences, Delhi Pharmaceutical Sciences and Research University, New Delhi-110017, India

Manvi Singh   Nanomedicine Laboratory, School of Pharmaceutical Education and Research, Jamia Hamdard, New Delhi-110062, India

Mohd. Aamir Mirza   Department of Pharmaceutics, Nanomedicine Laboratory, School of Pharmaceutical Education and Research, Jamia Hamdard, New Delhi-110062, India

Nazia Hassan   Nanomedicine Laboratory, School of Pharmaceutical Education and Research, Jamia Hamdard, New Delhi-110062, India

Pooja Jain   Nanomedicine Laboratory, School of Pharmaceutical Education and Research, Jamia Hamdard, New Delhi-110062, India

Rahmuddin Khan   Department of Pharmaceutics, Nanomedicine Laboratory, School of Pharmaceutical Education and Research, Jamia Hamdard, New Delhi-110062, India

Ranjita Misra   Sathyabama Institute of Science and Technology, Chennai-600119, Tamil Nadu, India

Sarita Kar   Department of Humanities and Social Sciences, Indian Institute of Technology (ISM) Dhandbad, Dhandbad-826004, Jharkhand, India

Salma Firdaus   Department of Pharmaceutics, School of Pharmaceutical Education and Research (SPER), Jamia Hamdard, New Delhi-110062, India

Sradhanjali Mohapatra   Department of Pharmaceutics, Nanomedicine Laboratory, School of Pharmaceutical Education and Research, Jamia Hamdard, New Delhi-110062, India

Uzma Farooq   Department of Pharmaceutics, Nanomedicine Laboratory, School of Pharmaceutical Education and Research, Jamia Hamdard, New Delhi-110062, India

Zeenat Iqbal   Department of Pharmaceutics, Nanomedicine Laboratory, School of Pharmaceutical Education and Research, Jamia Hamdard, New Delhi-110062, India

CHAPTER 1

Introduction to Cardiovascular Diseases and The Need for Nanomedicine and Regenerative Nanomedicine

Fahima Dilnawaz[1,*]

[1] *Laboratory of Nanomedicine, Institute of Life Sciences, Nalco Square, Chandrasekharpur, Bhubaneswar-751023, Odisha, India*

Abstract: Worldwide, cardiovascular diseases claim a number of lives; however, some of them are preventable with an early and proper management. Still, the treatment of cardiovascular diseases is limited as it deals with prescribed medicines administered orally and under critical condition with invasive surgery. Due to this, there exists an enormous gap in the area of medicine for the development of therapies for better patient outcomes. In this regard, recently, nanotechnological aspects of the development of medicines are sought, which may provide a solution for more effective treatment of disease, having better therapeutic outcomes with reduced side effect profile. Further, the regenerative nanomedicine therapeutic approach opens up a paradigm that deals with the repair of damaged heart tissue and future potential use of such systems.

Keywords: Bioavailability, Cardiomyocytes, Nanomaterials, Nanomedicine, Nanoscience.

INTRODUCTION

Cardiovascular diseases (CVDs) are one of the major causes of mortality and morbidity globally and include primarily hypertension and coronary artery diseases and their associated diseases like atherosclerosis, myocardial infarction, cardiac arrythmia, angina pectoris and chronic heart failure. CVDs are being accounted for the death of ~17.8 million people in 2017 and ~ 30% of all deaths occurring globally [1]. Of these deaths, around 7.3 million people died due to coronary artery disease and 6.2 million cases of deaths were due to stroke. Heart problems, which are often associated with reduced physical and mental health, lead to a decreased quality of life [2, 3]. Treatment for various CVDs includes

---

[*] **Corresponding author Fahima Dilnawaz:** Laboratory of Nanomedicine, Institute of Life Sciences, Nalco Square, Bhubanwswar-751023, Odisha, India; Tel: +91-674 – 2304341, E-mail: fahimadilnawaz@gmail.com

non-invasive therapy such as prescription medications and lifestyle modifications or invasive or surgical procedures such as bypass surgery, angioplasty *etc.*

During the past recent years, several advancements have been made in the field of diagnosis and treatment of various diseases with rapid expansion in nanoscience, which includes detailed molecular level understanding of diseases and use of sophisticated technologies in the nano range, in the field of medicine. Nanomedicine has emerged as a novel tool for the diagnosis and therapy of various Cardiovascular diseases [4]. National Institute of Health defines Nanomedicine as "the application of nanotechnological aspects for the diagnosis, treatment, monitoring and control of biological system." Nanotechnology is a collective term that refers to scaling down the particles to nanometer range (less than 1000 nm) [5]. The nanomaterials possess a relatively larger surface area compared to the same mass of materials, which makes the materials chemically reactive. Recent advances in nanoscience lead to the construction of new materials and devices that are used in molecular diagnostics and manufacturing of nanopharmaceuticals. These nanofeatured structures address the underlying cause of the cardiovascular disease that can improve the detection of early stage diseases so as to decrease premature mortality and enhance patient compliance for treatment [6, 7]. Nanomedicine serves to deliver a valuable set of research tools and clinical devices in the near future. Therapeutic delivery to the cardiovascular system may play an important role in the successful treatment of a variety of disease states, including atherosclerosis, ischemic-reperfusion injury and other types of microvascular diseases, including hypertension. Nanoformulated drugs are designed to protect against systemic degradation, thereby reducing toxicity, immunogenicity, and increasing half-life, bioavailability and precise biodistribution [4, 8]. Further to attain therapeutic selectivity to the heart, functionalization with targeting moieties allows specific accumulation in the diseased heart [6, 7]. In CVDs, thrombotic events occur in ischemic stroke, myocardial infarction, pulmonary embolism, and venous thrombosis, where thrombolytic therapy are used to break up the blood clots. Recombinant tissue plasminogen activator (tPA) is actively used as therapeutic molecule for the treatment of acute ischemic stroke [9]. Multifunctional nanoliposomes are used for highly specific binding to activated platelets whilst minimising undesirable side effects [10, 11]. Many nanoformulations are undergoing clinical trials; some are in the pipeline. CVN should be focused on disease-driven approach rather than formulation-driven approach to strengthen the significant potential and to overcome physiological barriers and improve therapeutic outcomes in patients. However, nanoformulation approach is still in infancy; great efforts are being made by the researchers for improved outcomes in the patients.

Regenerative nanomedicine emerged as another aspect of therapy where it demonstrates a considerable capacity for repairing damaged heart tissue [12]. As injuries to the heart are often permanent due to the limited proliferation and self-healing capability of cardiomyocytes [13]. In this regard, the development of patient specific cardiac cells is recognized as a useful strategy to overcome this problem. Engraftment of the therapeutic cells illustrates little turnout, due to cell rejection activity of the immune system. To overcome this, compatible biomaterials are used, which display exctracellular matrix activity (ECM). Stem cell based therapy has broad applications in cardiac regenerative medicine. To replenish the functional cells to the heart induced pluripotent stem cells (iPSC) and iPSC-derived cardiomyocytes (iCM) presents a better opportunity. The regenerative aspect of the cardiac cells can be further addressed with developed functional biomimetic engineered cardiac tissues through precise control over cell-cell and cell-ECM interactions can mimic the biological properties of the native environment in some way. The ongoing activities for cardiac regeneration are emerging fast and demonstrating promising outcome in preclinical studies [14].

Plasmonic nanoparticles for cardiovascular disease are quite specific and useful at different wavelengths of irradiation. These nanoparticles are responsive to various optical response and exhibit important changes which are strongly influenced by surface plasmon resonance (SPR) which are extremely useful in biomedical applications [15, 16]. The clinical application of nanomedicines in CVDs is currently under various clinical trials. Functional restoration of the vessel wall is very challenging; in this regard, nanoburning technique is implemented which can demolish and reverse the plaque, especially in combination with stem cell technology. In a 5 year clinical cohort study: nanomedicine in the real-world clinical practice, wherein, NANOM first-in-man trial was evaluated with an intention-to-treat population (nano *vs* ferro *vs* stenting) to demolish and reverse the plaque, especially in combination with stem cell for promising functional restoration of the vessel wall by the process of nanoburning. Outcome of this trial demonstrated high safety with a better rate of mortality, target lesion revascularization, major adverse cardiovascular events at the long-term follow-up when compared with everolimus drug eluting coronary stent XIENCE V® [17]. A clinical trial using gold nanoparticles with silica-iron oxide shells *versus* stenting was evaluated for the treatment of atherosclerosis. For which bioengineered structure NANOM-PCI was used, which effectively showed the ability for high-energy plasmonic photothermal burning under the near-infrared laser irradiation on the lesion and reduces the volume of the plaque with most optimal long term approach compared to stenting [18]. In the following section of chapters: **section -1**, we discuss various aspects of nanomedicinal approach towards CVDs along with ethical issues pertaining to it. In **section-2**: we discuss the regenerative cardiovascular nanomedicine.

CONSENT FOR PUBLICATION

Not Applicable.

CONFLICT OF INTEREST

The author confirms that this chapter contents have no conflict of interest.

ACKNOWLEDGEMENT

FD gratefully acknowledges the Dept. of Science and Technology, Govt. Of India, for the financial grant [SR/WOS-A/LS-448/2017 (G)] in the form of women scientist fellowship (WOS-A).

REFERENCES

[1]   Roth GA. Global, regional, and national age-sex-specific mortality for 282 causes of death in 195 countries and territories, 1980-2017: a systematic analysis for the Global Burden of Disease Study 2017. Lancet 2018; 392(10159): 1736-88.
        [http://dx.doi.org/10.1016/S0140-6736(18)32203-7] [PMID: 30496103]

[2]   Hobbs FD, Kenkre JE, Roalfe AK, Davis RC, Hare R, Davies MK. Impact of heart failure and left ventricular systolic dysfunction on quality of life: a cross-sectional study comparing common chronic cardiac and medical disorders and a representative adult population. Eur Heart J 2002; 23(23): 1867-76.
        [http://dx.doi.org/10.1053/euhj.2002.3255] [PMID: 12445536]

[3]   Juenger J, Schellberg D, Kraemer S, *et al.* Health related quality of life in patients with congestive heart failure: comparison with other chronic diseases and relation to functional variables. Heart 2002; 87(3): 235-41.
        [http://dx.doi.org/10.1136/heart.87.3.235] [PMID: 11847161]

[4]   Martín Giménez VM, Kassuha DE, Manucha W. Nanomedicine applied to cardiovascular diseases: latest developments. Ther Adv Cardiovasc Dis 2017; 11(4): 133-42.
        [http://dx.doi.org/10.1177/1753944717692293] [PMID: 28198204]

[5]   Sahoo SK, Parveen S, Panda JJ. The present and future of nanotechnology in human health care. Nanomedicine (Lond) 2007; 3(1): 20-31.
        [http://dx.doi.org/10.1016/j.nano.2006.11.008] [PMID: 17379166]

[6]   Lanza GM, Winter PM, Caruthers SD, *et al.* Nanomedicine opportunities for cardiovascular disease with perfluorocarbon nanoparticles. Nanomedicine (Lond) 2006; 1(3): 321-9.
        [http://dx.doi.org/10.2217/17435889.1.3.321] [PMID: 17716162]

[7]   Marsh JN, Senpan A, Hu G, *et al.* Fibrin-targeted perfluorocarbon nanoparticles for targeted thrombolysis. Nanomedicine (Lond) 2007; 2(4): 533-43.
        [http://dx.doi.org/10.2217/17435889.2.4.533] [PMID: 17716136]

[8]   Dormont F, Varna M, Couvreur P. Nanoplumbers: biomaterials to fight cardiovascular diseases. Mater Today 2018; 21(1): 122-43.
        [http://dx.doi.org/10.1016/j.mattod.2017.07.008]

[9]   Colasuonno M, Palange AL, Aid R, *et al.* Erythrocyte-inspired discoidal polymeric nanoconstructs

carrying tissue plasminogen activator for the enhanced lysis of blood clots. ACS Nano 2018; 12(12): 12224-37.
[http://dx.doi.org/10.1021/acsnano.8b06021] [PMID: 30427660]

[10]   Hsu HL, Chen JP. Preparation of thermosensitive magnetic liposome encapsulated recombinant tissue plasminogen activator for targeted thrombolysis. J Magn Magn Mater 2016; 427: 188-94.
[http://dx.doi.org/10.1016/j.jmmm.2016.10.122]

[11]   Huang Y, Yu L, Ren J, *et al.* An activated-platelet-sensitive nanocarrier enables targeted delivery of tissue plasminogen activator for effective thrombolytic therapy. J Control Release 2019; 300(28): 1-12.
[http://dx.doi.org/10.1016/j.jconrel.2019.02.033] [PMID: 30807804]

[12]   Cassani M, Fernandes S, Vrbsky J, Ergir E, Cavalieri F, Forte G. Combining nanomaterials and developmental pathways to design new treatments for cardiac regeneration: the pulsing heart of advanced therapies. Front Bioeng Biotechnol 2020; 6: 323-1-26.

[13]   Santoso MR, Ikeda G. Exosomes from induced pluripotent stem cell–derived cardiomyocytes promote autophagy for myocardial repair. J Am Heart Asso 2020; 9(6): e014345-1-14.

[14]   Dunn DA, Hodge AJ, Lipke EA. Biomimetic materials design for cardiac tissue regeneration. Wiley Interdiscip Rev Nanomed Nanobiotechnol 2014; 6(1): 15-39.
[http://dx.doi.org/10.1002/wnan.1241] [PMID: 24123919]

[15]   Liu J, He H, Xiao D, *et al.* Recent advances of plasmonic nanoparticles and their applications. Materials (Basel) 2018; 11(10): 1833.
[http://dx.doi.org/10.3390/ma11101833] [PMID: 30261657]

[16]   Kim M, Lee J-H, Nam J-M. Plasmonic photothermal nanoparticles for biomedical applications. Adv Sci (Weinh) 2019; 6(17)1900471
[http://dx.doi.org/10.1002/advs.201900471] [PMID: 31508273]

[17]   https://clinicaltrials.gov/ct2/show/NCT01270139

[18]   https://clinicaltrials.gov/ct2/show/NCT01436123

CHAPTER 2

Nanomedicinal Aspects in Cardiovascular Diseases

Uzma Farooq[1], Mohd. Aamir Mirza[1], Sradhanjali Mohapatra[1] and **Zeenat Iqbal[1,*]**

[1] *Nanomedicine Laboratory, Department of Pharmaceutics, School of Pharmaceutical Education and Research, Jamia Hamdard, New Delhi-110062, India*

Abstract: There is hardly any approved drug product for a cardiovascular ailment that utilizes nanotechnology. Although there are a few products in this category, they do not claim to be nano-therapeutics. An exhaustive evaluation of clinical trial databases indicates that in the near future, we may see some drug products in the market in this category. There are several similar investigational products by different groups across the globe. A comprehensive collection of published literature augurs the inclination of scientists in this field. The use of nanotechnology in cardiovascular is beneficial owing to Critical Quality Attributes that can be imparted based on the size, spatial arrangement of drug molecules, release profile, *etc*. In some cases, drug release characteristics have to be in sync with circadian rhythm, which can be easily obtained using this technology. The section of the book tries to highlight some of the aspects related to the exploration of nanotechnology in the case of cardiovascular treatment.

Keywords: Cardiac ischemia, CT, MRI, Nanomedicine, PET.

INTRODUCTION

According to the WHO's records, cardiovascular diseases are found to be the top most leading cause of death. Approximately 17.9 million people die every year worldwide due to the severity of cardiovascular disease and incurs (*i.e.* 31%) of all deaths. Out of these deaths, 85% are due to heart attack and stroke [1]. Annually by the year 2030, nearly 12 million deaths are expected to be caused by coronary atherosclerosis, which includes acute coronary syndromes like ST segment (*i.e* interval between ventricular depolarization and ventricular repolarization) or non ST segment elevation myocardial infarction. Cardiac ischemia might not reverse promptly; leading to the initiation of irreversible cell death, contractile dysfunction and scars tissue development [2].

---

[*] **Corresponding author Dr. Zeenat Iqbal:** Nanomedicine Laboratory, Department of Pharmaceutics, School of Pharmaceutical Education and Research (SPER), Jamia Hamdard, New Delhi-110062, India; Tel: +91-11-260586-9-5662, Fax: 011-26059663; E-mail: zeenatiqbal@jamiahamdard.ac.in

Despite the era of advanced technology in our scientific and clinical area, the death rate of heart diseases still remains high. Nanomedicine is the transitional science of nanotechnologies in healthcare, which involves the mechanism that leads to the development of new pathways at the molecular stage for the development of novel therapeutics and diagnosis of cardiovascular disease (CVDs) [3]. Nanomedicine has various applications in therapeutics; nanotechnologies such as nanoemulsions, nanoparticles or nanodevices are used to penetrate the biological barriers. The nano-devices can contain encapsulated active molecules for the locoregional delivery of the targeted area. These are also used to cross the biological barrier for the systemic effect [4]. The advance of treatment modalities include pharmaceuticals, reconstitution by surgery and implantation of devices. Although these conventional treatment technologies provide a better quality of life but still needs improvement in therapeutics, or else it requires other alternative therapeutic approaches. Recent technologies of nanostructured systems, nanomedicines, nanoscience and nanotechnology have provided unique properties that can potentially overcome the limitations of conventional cardiovascular pharmaceutical medicines through the development of novel pharmaceutical nanomedicines and biomedical devices. Bioengineering perspective towards the diagnosis of atherosclerosis and other cardiac disorder provides exclusive opportunities for the diagnostic and management of these disorders. Further, studies on molecular engineering have provided new pathways that can potentially serve for diagnostic and therapeutic targeted delivery **(Fig. 1)**.

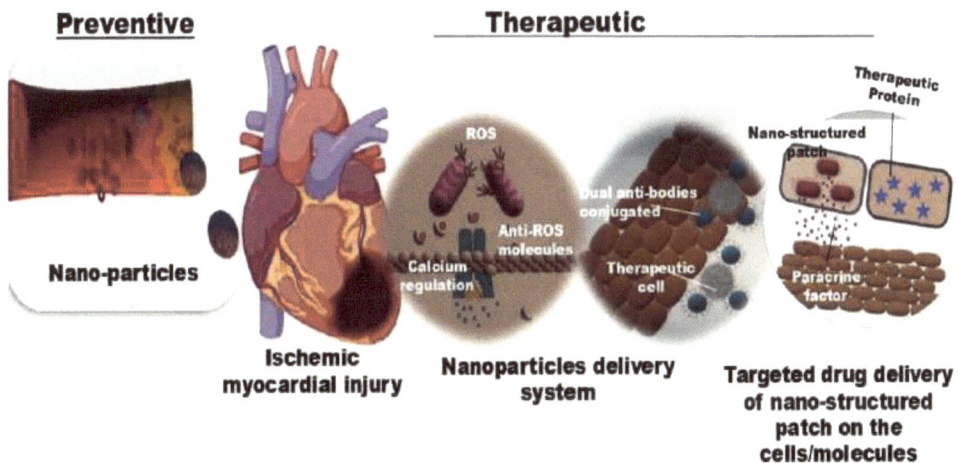

Fig. (1). Nanoparticles or nanostructured biomaterials can be used for delivery of cells and molecules and for targeted therapy of artherosclerosis or Ischaemic myocardial injury.

Radiotracers images obtained by various nuclear imaging techniques, such as single-photon emission computed tomography (SPECT) and positron emission, respectively (PET), are used to determine the cardiac disorder *via* exogenous administration whereas, for the anatomical imaging of arteries, advanced nanomedicine techniques are used including magnetic resonance imaging (MRI), ultrasonography (US) and computed tomography (CT) [5]. Drugs are commonly delivered either *via* oral route or needle based routes, such as intramuscular, intravenous or subcutaneous, which are painful for the patients. In the current technology platform, nanoparticles can be administered *via* intranasal route to treat cardiac disorder. As we know, inhalational delivery is a common route for a respiratory disorder. In one study, peptide –loaded nanoparticles are administered *via* inhalation for cardiac targeted therapy [6]. This study, reported that inhalation therapy is suitable for carrying peptide based nanoformulation to the cardiac disorder as it deals with biomineralized inspired technique without any toxic effect and lacks interference in the functional activity of the cardiac myocytes. For imaging aspect, nanoparticles are formulated with the contrast agent that are either attached on the particles surface, or encapsulated with fluorescent dyes in the matrix or a combination of both.

ADVANCES OF NANOMEDICINE FOR DIAGNOSIS OF CVDS

Vascular physiology under normal condition was found to be tight (< 2 nm) junction of endothelial membrane, which is responsible for preventing the penetration of nanoformulations. However, endothelial dysfunction creates gap in-between the cells, which enables the microparticles or nanoparticles to penetrate from the blood vessels at topical sites, in turn, unabling to get cleared owing to its lymphatic impairment. Development of contrast generating nanomaterials for the use of radioactive imaging, fluorescent, para/super-paramagnetic, LSP (light scattering particles) and electron dense method were sought by combining multiple contrast agents at nanoscale for the detection and analysis of cardiovascular disorders at an early stage. MRI for cardiovascular imaging requires powerful magnetic fields or radiofrequency waves for the diagnosis *via* internal structures scanning. The size dependent imaging properties of fluorescent nanoparticles enable the detection level from ultraviolet to mid-infrared range and its enhancement of emission wavelength are correlated with the particle size [7]. These multistage nanoparticles provide images of the target areas where macrophages are accumulated. Nanocontrast agents like ^{18}F-CLIO (^{18}F-cross linking with iron oxide) are used for the detection with PET and MRI. Three iron oxide nanoformulations such as AMI-121 (Ferumoxsil^{TM}); OMP50 and AMI-25 (Feridex) are approved for imaging by FDA [7].

NANOPARTICLES FOR MRI

Various types of contrast agent, such as inorganic metal oxide having limited transverse relaxation time are used for signal enhancement in MRI imaging. Super-paramagnetic iron oxide and gadolinium have the ability to reduce the relaxation time of tissues longitudinally and to enhance the strength of signals for positive contrast [8]. Therefore, nanocrystal of magnetic moment and hydrophilic core exposure is responsible for determining the intensity of signal.

NANOPARTICLES FOR POSITRON EMITTING TOMOGRAPHY (PET)

PET imaging is suggestively used to determine the variation in the anatomical, physiological, functional changes in transmitted signals in the cardiovascular system. PET provides high sensitive images due to the radiation emitted from radiopharmaceutical that is being injected to patients intravenously. These radiotracers suffer short half-lives and are also toxic to tissues. In order to overcome these issues, multi-imaging nanoparticles were designed by incorporating Quantum dots (QD), super-paramagnetic iron oxide nanoparticles or gold nanoparticles. Surface of the nanoparticles is coated with radioligand chelate *i.e.* capable of introducing PET imaging [9].

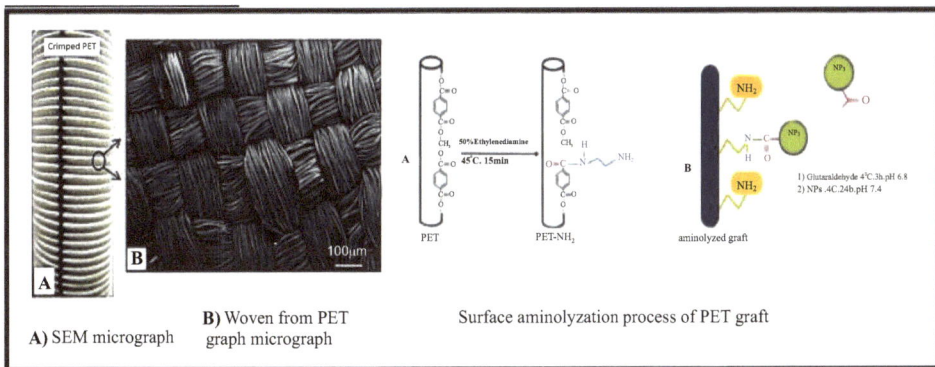

Fig. (2). Immobilization and characterization of PLGA nanoparticles on polyethylene terephthalate cardiovascular grafts for local drug therapy of associated graft complication: reused with kind permission of authors of another study [22].

For coronary atherosclerosis, biodegradable nanoparticles are designed for therapeutic delivery of biomolecules to the targeted area, which can control the plaques by reducing inflammation *via* activation of pro-resolving pathways or removing crystals of lipids and cholesterol. To reduce the inflammation, biodegradable polymeric material will be able to release the encapsulated biomolecules or proteins in a controlled manner. A membrane receptor (CD163) can be used for imaging of CD163 expression macrophages in order to detect atherosclerosis plague [10]. Tarin *et al.* designed a targeted probe based on gold-coated iron oxide nanoparticles conjugated with anti-CD163. Results demonstrated that these developed nanoparticles are highly sensitive and capable of detecting CD163 expression which in turn can provide useful information regarding the disorder [11]. In another study, superparamagnetic nanosilica@ PLGA nanoparticle loaded quercetin are formulated for the treatment of heart failure, myocardial infarction, coronary cardiac disease, atherosclerosis and inflammatory heart disease and other related CVDs. Widest health problems across the globe includes unhealthy diet, sedentary lifestyle, various other diseases like obesity that leads to many CVDs can be preventable and few can be treated with the help of the nanoformulations (Fig. **3**).

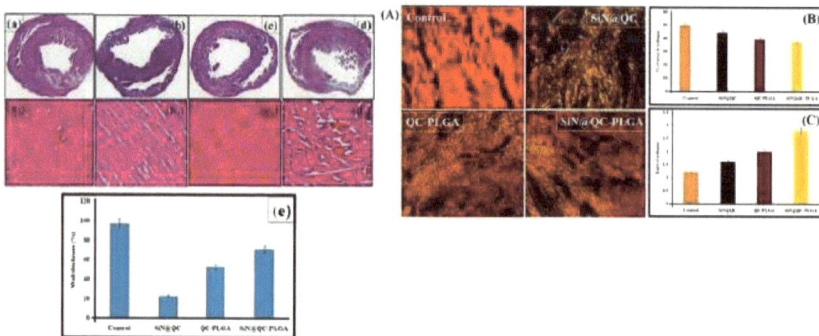

Fig. (3). Fabrication and characterization of superparamagnetic nano-silica of quercetin-encapsulated PLGA nanoformulation: Effect on rat cardio after 1month of treatment observed by hematoxylin and eosin (H&E) staining which shows significantly widening of left ventricle. Effect on rat cardio after 1month treatment observed by PSR staining [24].

Moreover, CVDs remained the leading cause of death, in which the mortality rate has been steadily increased and even crossed the statistics of cancer. Currently, the treatment of CVDs is revolved around the oral medications, lifestyle alteration and invasive surgery. Hence, this area demands intervention of newer technology. Nanomedicine, which is among the fastest emerging area of medical research is expected to provide a greater potential and effective treatment approach with fewer side effects. Various experiments have been conducted which are focused on cardiovascular applications, but very few of them have entered the clinical trials Table **1**

Nanotechnology can be exploited for the early detection and treatment of several diseases. Based on the classification of antihypertensive drugs, angiotensin converting enzyme inhibitors such as enalapril, captopril, ramipril are mostly administered to prevent the conversion of angiotensin I into angiotensin II [16]. These administered drugs incur various adverse effect such as limited bioavailability, permeability, which in turn demands high frequency of dosing. In this regard, nanotechnology based formulations have provided an alternative strategy for resolving related problems as well as challenges. Drugs like digitalis or digoxin are generally administered in acute myocardial infarction and arrhythmia to increase the transmitted signal for normalizing the heart function. HMG-CoA reductase inhibitor inhibits the action of enzyme, which is responsible to transfer HMG-CoA into mevalonic acid for the synthesis of cholesterol [17]. The main objective of using nanotechnology in pharmacy is to treat the patient effectively and efficiently with increased patient compliance. Formulated nanodrugs are intended to prevent adverse side effects by introducing ligand-targeting, receptor-mediated targeting or stimuli-responsive targeting approaches, that might provide an additional strategy for implementation of localized release of the loaded drug for better use in diagnostics, molecular imaging and tissue engineering *etc* [18]. The following table provides brief information of recent advances of nanomedicine formulations developed by using various evaluation parameters for early diagnosis and treatment of cardiovascular disorders (Table **2**), and brief idea about the development of technologies up-till now as well as patents related to advancement of nanomedicine (Table **3**).

Table 1. Clinical trials (CT) data on the advanced technologies of nanomedicine for the treatment of CVDs.

SL No	CT No	Title of The Study	Interventions	References
1	NCT03659864	The role of eicosanoids in the cardiovascular actions of inhaled nanoparticles	Carbon nanoparticles were found among diesel exhaust particulate, filtering air small and ultrasmall graphene oxide	[12]
2	NCT03083717	Application of nanotechnology and chemical sensors for the diagnosis of decompensated heart failure by respiratory samples	Analysis of exhaled breath for the diagnosis *via* nano-material-based sensors (NaNose)	[13]
3	IRCT201610271083N8	The impact of synthesis of bio-Nano materials in acceleration blood clotting	Administration of bio-Nano materials in angiography area until it completely prevented coagulation and bleeding using specified clinical procedure	[14]
4	NCT03719079	The nanowear wearable heart failure management system multiple-sensor algorithm (Nanosense)	Development and validation trial with the nanosense data collection study to predict worsening heart failure	[15]

Table 2. List investigated nano-formulations used for various indications of CVDs along with different evaluation parameters for analysis.

S. No.	Nano Material of CVS	Indication	Reference
2.	Nanoparticle-eluting stents design by a cationic electro-deposition coating technology	A bio-absorbable polymeric nanoparticles-eluting stent for the efficient and prolonged delivery on the cardiovascular disease	[19]
3.	Nanoparticles containing the pro-resolving peptide Ac2-26 against atherosclerosis.	The therapeutic efficacy of pro-resolving peptide Ac2-26 loaded nano-particles for targeted delivery in the atherosclerosis lesions.	[20]
4.	Multi-phase nano-emulsion of arbutin and coumaric acid as bioactive components	Nano-emulsion effectively co-deliver hydrophilic arbutin and hydrophobic coumaric acid for the improvement of bio-accessibility nutraceuticals essential phenolic compounds. Lactobacillus beverage was also used to determine the suitability of nutraceuticals incorporating nano-emulsion	[21]
5.	PLGA nanoparticles were covalently immobilized on to the woven form of crimped polyethylene terephthalate (PET,Dacron®) cardiovascular graft for local drug therapy	Immobilized nanoparticles manifested stability under blood flow-mimetic conditions for 24h. it was used to treat the early thrombosis, inflammation, or bacterial infection *via* local delivery of therapeutic agents.	[22]
6.	3D printed PLA biodegradable polymeric stent	The heparinized 3D printed PLA stent provides a promising clinical strategy to avoid vascular stent associated complications.	[23]
7.	Super-paramagnetic nano-silica@quercetin encapsulated PLGA nano-composite.	A novel nanobiocomposite was created so as to improve poor watery solvency and steadiness of the medication with the point of preventing atherosclerosis and articulation of heart proteins.	[24]
8.	Nano-emulsified gamma-oryzanol	Nano-emulsion (NEORY) confers better results of hyper-cholesterolaemia, oxidative stress and heart weight, as well as regulation of hepatic transcriptional cholesterol metabolism	[25]
9	Nanoparticle eluting angioplasty balloons	acrylic-based hydrogel (AAH) coated nanoparticles illustrated better transfer efficiency or local delivery of anti-restenosis drugs directly to the injured arteries after angioplasty	[26]
10	Meta-tetra(hydroxyphenyl) chlorine loaded polymeric micelles	The AAH coating of drug-loaded NPs on the angioplasty balloon could potentially provide superior retention of drug-loaded NPs on to the arterial wall for a better local delivery of drug-loaded NPs to effectively treat arterial diseases	[27]
11.	Electrospun nanofibres	Used for investigating *in-vitro* PROP release of drug from uniaxial and coaxial nano-fibers prepared by electro-spinning	[28]

Table 3. List investigated nano-formulations used for various indications of CVDs along with different evaluation parameters for analysis.

S.No	Nano–Medicinal Technology	Invention	Action	References
1	Targeted SNO-nan--fibers US9517275B2	Targeted drug delivery to prevent restenosis in the cardiovascular system	Inhibition of neointimal hyperplasia by the targeted SNO-Nanofiber	[29]
2	Stimulus responsive nanocomplexes, WO2014/197816A1	Comprises of a therapeutic agent and a masking moiety that prevents the therapeutic agent from exerting its biological activity.	Heparin-Peptide Nano-complexes, which do not prolong clotting time, do not increase bleeding, prevents thrombosis *in vivo* .	[30]
3	coated cerium oxide (CeO2) particles *via* nano-encapsulation, WO2014/153160A2	multi-layered encapsulation of cerium oxide particles is useful for enhancing their anti-oxidative activity, maximization of potent antioxidant's biocompatibility, increase in particles' target cell penetration and uptake, reduction of off-target effects and retention of high anti-oxidative activity.	Demonstrate the effectiveness of inhaled nanoparticles in an animal model of emphysema, of Parkinson 's Disease	[31]
4	Nanofibrous scaffold comprising immobilized cells US8691543B2	The two part polyurethane scaffold device prevents migration of human mesenchymal stem cells (hMSCs) and allows communication between the stem cells and native cardiomyocytes and seals the gap junction formation through pores for minimally invasive delivery.	Used for gap junction assay and determination of protein diffusion across the membrane	[32]

CONCLUSION

Applications of nanotechnology in medicine, particularly in cardiovascular disease offers incredible therapeutic promise. Nanotechnology has offered sustained release activity; prolong circulation, specific delivery and imaging ability by circumventing many limitations of the traditional therapy for the treatment of numerous CVDs. These developments are only the beginning of tremendous future growth that lies ahead for CVDs.

CONSENT FOR PUBLICATION

Not Applicable.

CONFLICT OF INTEREST

The author confirms that this chapter contents have no conflict of interest.

ACKNOWLEDGEMENT

Declared none.

REFERENCES

[1]   https://www.who.int/health-topics/cardiovascular-diseases

[2]   Rezende PC, Ribas FF, Serrano CV Jr, Hueb W. Clinical significance of chronic myocardial ischemia in coronary artery disease patients. J Thorac Dis 2019; 11(3): 1005-15.
[http://dx.doi.org/10.21037/jtd.2019.02.85] [PMID: 31019790]

[3]   Chandarana M, Curtis A, Hoskins C. The use of nanotechnology in cardiovascular disease. Appl Nanosci 2018; 8: 1607-19.
[http://dx.doi.org/10.1007/s13204-018-0856-z]

[4]   Weltring MK, Gouze N, Martin N, Pereira N, Baanante I, Gramatica F. Strategic Research and Innovation Agenda For Nanomedicine. https://etp-nanomedicineeu/2016; 1-31.

[5]   Sanz J, Fayad ZA. Imaging of atherosclerotic cardiovascular disease. Nature 2008; 451(7181): 953-7.
[http://dx.doi.org/10.1038/nature06803] [PMID: 18288186]

[6]   Miragoli M, Ceriotti P, Iafisco M, *et al.* Inhalation of peptide-loaded nanoparticles improves heart failure. Sci Transl Med 2018; 10(424)eaan6205
[http://dx.doi.org/10.1126/scitranslmed.aan6205] [PMID: 29343624]

[7]   Bejarano J, Navarro-Marquez M, Morales-Zavala F, *et al.* Nanoparticles for diagnosis and therapy of atherosclerosis and myocardial infarction: evolution toward prospective theranostic approaches. Theranostics 2018; 8(17): 4710-32.
[http://dx.doi.org/10.7150/thno.26284] [PMID: 30279733]

[8]   Eriksson P, Tal AA, Skallberg A, *et al.* Cerium oxide nanoparticles with antioxidant capabilities and gadolinium integration for MRI contrast enhancement. Sci Rep 2018; 8(1): 6999.
[http://dx.doi.org/10.1038/s41598-018-25390-z] [PMID: 29725117]

[9]   Savla R, Minko T. Nanoparticle design considerations for molecular imaging of apoptosis: Diagnostic, prognostic, and therapeutic value. Adv Drug Deliv Rev 2017; 113: 122-40.
[http://dx.doi.org/10.1016/j.addr.2016.06.016] [PMID: 27374457]

[10]   Mulder WJ, Jaffer FA, Fayad ZA, Nahrendorf M. Imaging and nanomedicine in inflammatory atherosclerosis. Sci Transl Med 2014; 6(239)239sr1
[http://dx.doi.org/10.1126/scitranslmed.3005101] [PMID: 24898749]

[11]   Tarin C, Carril M, Martin-Ventura JL, *et al.* Targeted gold-coated iron oxide nanoparticles for CD163 detection in atherosclerosis by MRI. Sci Rep 2015; 5: 17135.
[http://dx.doi.org/10.1038/srep17135] [PMID: 26616677]

[12]   https://clinicaltrials.gov/ct2/show/NCT03659864

[13]   https://clinicaltrials.gov/ct2/show/NCT03083717

[14]   https://en.irct.ir/trial/105

[15]   https://clinicaltrials.gov/ct2/history/NCT0371907

[16]   Martín Giménez VM, Kassuha DE, Manucha W. Nanomedicine applied to cardiovascular diseases: latest developments. Ther Adv Cardiovasc Dis 2017; 11(4): 133-42.
[http://dx.doi.org/10.1177/1753944717692293] [PMID: 28198204]

[17]   Park JH, Dehaini D, Zhou J, Holay M, Fang RH, Zhang L. Biomimetic nanoparticle technology for cardiovascular disease detection and treatment. Nanoscale Horiz 2020; 5(1): 25-42.
[http://dx.doi.org/10.1039/C9NH00291J] [PMID: 32133150]

[18]   Iafisco M, Alogna A, Miragoli M, Catalucci D. Nanomedicine (Lond) 2019; 14(8): 1-4.
[PMID: 30548078]

[19]   Nakano K, Egashira K, Masuda S, *et al.* Formulation of nanoparticle-eluting stents by a cationic electrodeposition coating technology: efficient nano-drug delivery *via* bioabsorbable polymeric nanoparticle-eluting stents in porcine coronary arteries. JACC Cardiovasc Interv 2009; 2(4): 277-83.
[http://dx.doi.org/10.1016/j.jcin.2008.08.023] [PMID: 19463437]

[20]   Fredman G, Kamaly N, Spolitu S, *et al.* Targeted nanoparticles containing the proresolving peptide Ac2-26 protect against advanced atherosclerosis in hypercholesterolemic mice. Sci Transl Med 2015; 7(275)275ra20
[http://dx.doi.org/10.1126/scitranslmed.aaa1065] [PMID: 25695999]

[21]   Huang H, Belwal T, Liu S, Duan Z, Luo Z. Novel multi-phase nano-emulsion preparation for co-loading hydrophilic arbutin and hydrophobic coumaric acid using hydrocolloids. Food Hydrocoll 2019; 93: 92-101.
[http://dx.doi.org/10.1016/j.foodhyd.2019.02.023]

[22]   Al Meslmani BM, Mahmoud GF, Bakowsky U. Immobilization and characterization of PLGA nanoparticles on polyethylene terephthalate cardiovascular grafts for local drug therapy of associated graft complications. J Drug Deliv Sci Technol 2018; 47: 144-50.
[http://dx.doi.org/10.1016/j.jddst.2018.07.011]

[23]   Lee SJ, Jo HH, Lim KS, Lim D, Lee S, Lee JH, *et al.* Heparin coating on 3d printed poly (l-lactic acid) biodegradable cardiovascular stent *via* mild surface modification approach for coronary artery implantation. Chem Eng J 2019; 378122116
[http://dx.doi.org/10.1016/j.cej.2019.122116]

[24]   Wang L, Feng M, Li Y, *et al.* Fabrication of superparamagnetic nano-silica@ quercetin-encapsulated PLGA nanocomposite: Potential application for cardiovascular diseases. J Photochem Photobiol B 2019; 196111508
[http://dx.doi.org/10.1016/j.jphotobiol.2019.05.005] [PMID: 31152936]

[25]   Ishaka A, Imam MU, Ismail M, *et al.* Nanoemulsified gamma-oryzanol rich fraction blend regulates hepatic cholesterol metabolism and cardiovascular disease risk in hypercholesterolaemic rats. J Funct Foods 2016; 26: 338-49.
[http://dx.doi.org/10.1016/j.jff.2016.08.015]

[26]   Iyer R, Kuriakose AE, Yaman S, *et al.* Nanoparticle eluting-angioplasty balloons to treat cardiovascular diseases. Int J Pharm 2019; 554: 212-23.
[http://dx.doi.org/10.1016/j.ijpharm.2018.11.011] [PMID: 30408532]

[27]   Wennink JWH, Liu Y, Mäkinen PI, *et al.* Macrophage selective photodynamic therapy by meta-tetra(hydroxyphenyl)chlorin loaded polymeric micelles: A possible treatment for cardiovascular diseases. Eur J Pharm Sci 2017; 107: 112-25.
[http://dx.doi.org/10.1016/j.ejps.2017.06.038] [PMID: 28679107]

[28]   Oliveira MF, Suarez D, Rocha JC, *et al.* Electrospun nanofibers of polyCD/PMAA polymers and their potential application as drug delivery system. Mater Sci Eng C 2015; 54: 252-61.
[http://dx.doi.org/10.1016/j.msec.2015.04.042] [PMID: 26046289]

[29]   Kibbe MR, Stupp SI, Moyer TJ. https://patentsgooglecom/patent/US201501510022016; 1-35.

[30]   Yu-ming Lin K, Bhatia SN, Kwong GA, *et al.* Stimulus responsive nanocomplexes and methods of use thereof US20140364368A1. Massachusetts Institute of Technology 2014; pp. 1-14.

[31]   Leiter J, Gillmor S, Jeremic A, Vert-Wong E, Fairbrothers G. Fairbrothers G. Method of enhancing the biodistribution and tissue targeting properties of thera peutic ce02 particles *via* nano-encapsulation and coating. WO2014153160A2 2014; 1-95.

[32]   Gaudette G, Phaneuf MD, Ali S, Almeida B, Alfonzo H, Flynn K. Nanofibrous scaffold comprising immobilized cells US8691543B2. Worcester Polytechnic Institute Biosurfaces Inc. 2014; pp. 1-24.

CHAPTER 3

Role of Nanomedicine in the Diagnosis of Cardiovascular Diseases

Foziyah Zakir[1,2]**, Mohd. Aamir Mirza**[1]**, Rahmuddin Khan**[1] **and Zeenat Iqbal**[1,*]

[1] *Nanomedicine Laboratory, Department of Pharmaceutics, School of Pharmaceutical Education & Research, Jamia Hamdard, New Delhi-110062, India*

[2] *Department of Pharmaceutics, School of Pharmaceutical Sciences, Delhi Pharmaceutical Sciences and Research University, New Delhi-110017, India*

Abstract: Various lifestyle related factors are primarily responsible for the increase of cardiovascular diseases. The development of numerous diseases such as acute myocardial infarction, stroke and thrombosis need multiple therapies. These therapies are based on synthetic active ingredients, which in long-term usage, give adverse side effects. Currently, a lot of attention has been focused on nanotechnology based drug formulation, which can provide sustained drug release, increased half-life, and in turn, can circumvent limitations of conventional therapies. With the advent of the nanomedical approach, the survival length of the patients can be prolonged. This chapter mostly focuses on widely used nanomedicines in therapy and imaging of cardiovascular diseases.

Keywords: Dendrimers, Liposomes, Micelles, Nanocarrier, Nanomedicine, Polymeric.

INTRODUCTION

Cardiovascular diseases (CVDs) are one of the prominent reasons for the death of millions of lives. It is reported by WHO that cardiovascular complications claimed 17.7 million deaths in 2015 and the number is estimated to rise to 23.6 million by 2030 [1]. Dietary factors such as high intake of salt, sugar, saturated fat-rich diet as well as sedentary lifestyle increase the chances of CVD. Some other well-known contributors to the disease are genetic predisposition, age, diabetes, stress and obesity. With the disappearance of traditional cultures such as the consumption of organic food, stress-free life and heavy physical activity, the incidence of CVD is on the rise. Nevertheless, the epidemic, although declining in

* **Corresponding author Dr. Zeenat Iqbal** Nanomedicine Laboratory, Department of Pharmaceutics, School of Pharmaceutical Education & Research, Jamia Hamdard, New Delhi-110062, India; Tel: +91-11-26058689-5662, Fax: 011-26059663, E-mail: zeenatiqbal@jamiahamdard.ac.in

Fahima Dilnawaz and Zeenat Iqbal (Eds.)

developed countries, is growing in developing countries. CVDs are a pool of heart diseases comprising congestive heart failure, coronary cardiac failure, myocardial infarction, inflammatory heart disease, deep vein thrombosis, *etc.* that result in tissue death and, eventually, mortality.

The rising numbers of statistics clearly indicate the need for newer treatments and technological developments to fight CVDs. The first stage in the pathogenesis of CVD complications is atherosclerosis. Atherosclerosis is the hardening of fat, cholesterol, calcium or macrophage cells overtime to form plaques. These plaques, which get deposited in the vasculature, result in congestion that severely hampers the blood flow and, in severe cases, it can even rupture the blood vessels leading to ischemia [2]. The introduction and approval of coronary stents by the US FDA in 1994 have seen major breakthroughs in the area. Other surgical methods, including bypass surgery and angioplasty even though can be modified for refinement but their efficiency is still questionable. Decades later, medicine still relies upon 'blockbuster' therapies such as beta-adrenergic blocking agents, diuretics and HMG-CoA reductase inhibitors for the treatment of vascular diseases. These treatments aim at reducing the build-up in the blood vessels and restore normal blood flow. Again, these drugs also present shortcomings such as significant adverse effects, poor response and lack of patient compliance [3]. Nanotechnology could be a promising potential for the delivery of drugs and genes for the management of cardiovascular problems (Fig. **1**).

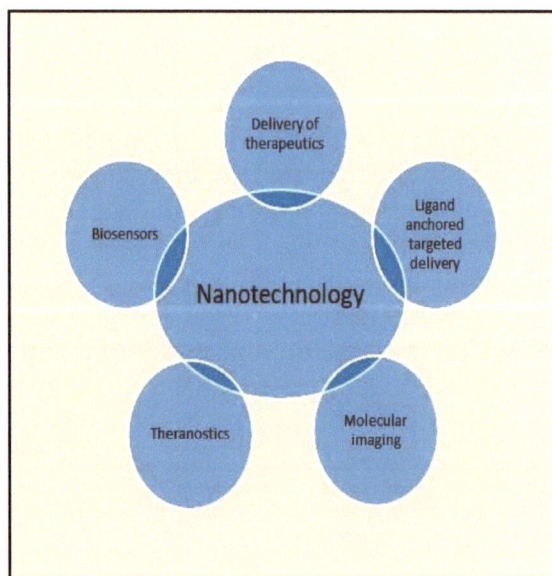

Fig. (1). Applications of nanotechnology in cardiovascular medicine.

Combination therapies encompassing delivery of multidrug in the same carrier are becoming increasingly popular. The various advancements in nanotechnology have led to reduced toxicity, reduced side effects and prolonged delivery of drugs [4]. Additionally, the technology can also be used to improve the performance of cardiac stents by providing nanomaterial coating or controlled release of therapeutics. The area of nanotechnology has also witnessed advances in target-specific molecular imaging. The early identification of a CVD is very crucial as it helps improve prognosis. Targeting can be achieved either through conjugation of a therapeutic molecule to a ligand or by coupling with a high molecular weight polymer that will enhance the penetration in vascular tissues [5]. These include liposomes, micelles, polymeric nanoparticles, dendrimers [6], *etc.,* which will be explained in detail in the following section. The different delivery systems used in nanotechnology have been figuratively detailed (Fig. **2**).

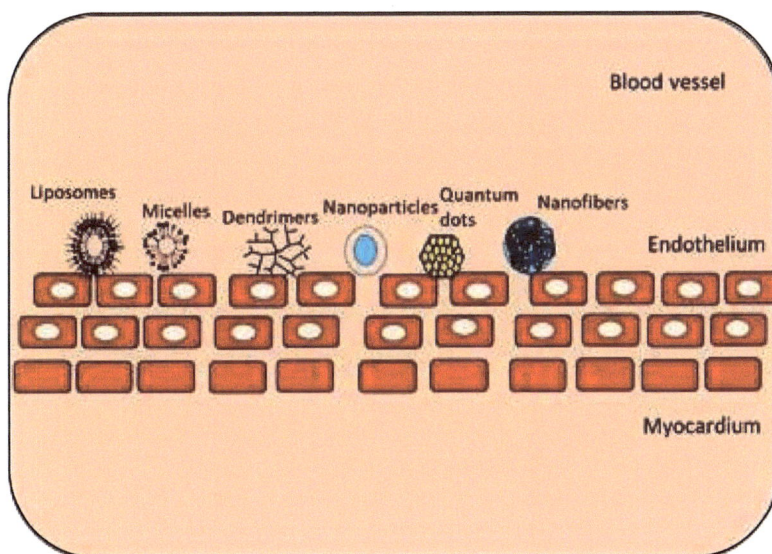

Fig. (2). The various nanodelivery systems used for the treatment of cardiovascular complications.

LIPOSOMES

Liposomes are essential vesicles, made up of phospholipids and cholesterol in their outer layers surrounding the hydrophilic core in sizes of 50-200 nm [7]. The delivery system can be used for the encapsulation of both lyophobic and lyophilic drugs. The type of liposome is small or large unilamellar vesicles and multilamellar vesicles are small-sized single lipid bilayer vesicles, large-sized single lipid bilayer vesicles or multiple layered bilayer vesicles, respectively affect the drug loading [8]. Therapeutic delivery of CVD drugs faces a number of challenges such as short half-lives, lack of control on drug release, non-specific distribution, thus advocates the use of high concentrations of drugs leading to adverse side effects. The liposome technology remedies these obstacles by providing controlled release and the possibility of targeting the desired action area. Additionally, it also improves the residence time, protects the drug from degradation whilst preventing toxicity. The liposome technology has been used for the delivery of various drugs to improve therapeutic efficacy and bioavailability. Recently, alendronate loaded liposomes are underway in phase II clinical trial to determine their ability to reduce restenosis in patients. Delivery of genetic material by liposome technology, generally known as lipoplexes, has been gaining wide attention for the treatment of CVDs. For instance, transport of metalloproteinase-1 inhibitor was facilitated by liposomes and significant recovery in vascular injury was observed [9]. In another study, 90 cDNA was transfected by liposomes in chronic ischemia rabbit model followed by improved perfusion [10]. These studies indicate liposomes can be used as an alternate to viral vectors for transfection. A hybrid vector commonly used is the hemagglutinating virus of Japan (HVJ) liposome. Inactivated HVJ is complexed with liposomes encapsulating genetic material. The virus is a complex of neuraminidase and fusion proteins which facilitate transfection of a gene into the cytoplasm [11].

Targeting can be achieved by manipulating the surface of liposomes using techniques such as PEGylation where PEG is coupled to the surface to impart hydrophilicity to the carrier system with the aim to prolong circulation. The concept is better known as stealth liposomes [12]. Furthermore, other targeting moieties and antibodies can be attached to the surface for specific delivery [13]. In this regard platelet, targeted liposomes have been gaining popularity because of their potential in atherosclerosis, myocardial infarction and thrombosis. Urokinase, which is a thrombolytic drug, has been encapsulated in liposomes and functionalized with arginyl-glycyl-aspartic acid (cRGD) peptide which has the potential to target GPIIb/IIIa receptors present on platelet surface [14]. Further, liposomes can also be used for targeting the blood vessels. The endothelial cells present on the surface of vessel walls act as a good target because of their close proximity to the blood. The various endothelial adhesion molecules such as ICAM-1 [15], selectins [16] and integrins [17] have been explored for active targeting of liposomes bearing therapeutic agent and coupled with site-specific ligands. Another area in cardiovascular research is a diagnosis where liposomes have shown promising potential. Liposomes loaded with ^{99}m-Tc-radiolabelled enzymes [18], streptokinase [19] and urokinase [20] have demonstrated improved uptake by thrombus and useful for the diagnosis of thrombosis. Anti-ICAM-1 conjugated to PEGylated liposomes preloaded with iohexol have shown potential in the detection of atherosclerotic plaques [21]. Similarly, the capability to bind to endothelial cells has been explored by PEGylated liposomes loaded with Gadolinium-diethylenetriaminepentaacetic acid-bis(stearyl amide), which has been used as a diagnostic tool [22]. Adiponectin coupled with liposomes have been investigated as an imaging tool for atherosclerotic plaques. *Ex-vivo* studies have shown strong fluorescence on the surface of plaques on treatment with the delivery system [23]. Recently Fumagillin loaded liposomes were tested for their anti-angiogenic efficacy in atherosclerotic lesions and a significant decrease in lesion sizes in the mice model was observed [24]. In spite of vast research, none of the liposomal formulations are available in the market which stresses the need for further research to improve the therapeutic efficacy and liposomal stability.

POLYMERIC NANOPARTICLES

Nanotechnology has significant applications in CVD owing to its high surface area to volume ratio, high surface area and increased surface activity which ultimately leads to wettability and better interaction between nanomaterials and tissue at the molecular level [25]. Nanoparticles act as a drug carrier with the ability to cross the endothelium of blood vessels. The nanoparticles have the advantage of uptake by myocardial cells with limited possibility for embolization. Additionally, functionalization can target the drug molecule to the desired area. The nanoparticulate technology has also been explored for the diagnosis of CVDs such as for the diagnosis of atherosclerosis. Magnetic nanoparticles were prepared for sensing vascular cell adhesion molecule-1, which is an inflammation indicator [26]. In another study, ultrasmall superparamagnetic iron oxide particles coated with dextran were used for the detection of the rejection site of cardiac allograft [27]. Recently, theranostic nanoparticles have come into foreplay which combines imaging and therapeutic applications. One of the successful studies in this area is the use of fluorescent nanoparticles coated with dextran to target plaque macrophages. The photosensitizer showed the capability to detect and kill macrophages which is useful in atherosclerosis therapy [28].

NANOTECHNOLOGY IN BIOMATERIALS

An interesting application of nanotechnology is its ability to expand the functional and biological properties of various cardiovascular devices [29]. More recently, nanostructure surface have wide potential in cardiovascular medicine. The various techniques to produce nanostructures are chemical etching [30], photolithography [31], capillary force lithography [32], direct writing [33] and anodization [34]. In this regard various metal nanoparticles have been explored. For instance, magnesium oxide nanoparticles are widely used due to its anti-bacterial properties [35]. Similarly, it has been reported hydroxyapatite nanoparticles could improve protein absorption [36]. The unique feature of gold nanoparticles is their stability against chemical reactions, which make them an attractive substrate for functionalization. In one such study, gold nanoparticles were fabricated to release nitric oxide, which acts as a mediator of vascular smooth muscle functions [37]. The various applications are improved cellular uptake, targeting cells, delivery of drugs or genes and diagnosis [38]. Polymeric nanoparticles are more favoured because of their tunable properties. In one of the works, PLGA was immobilized on PTFE films to produce vascular grafts [39]. Nanocomposites are composed of metal, polymeric or ceramic matrix materials with a functional component in nanosize. Some of the examples are polyurethane nanocomposites for the fabrication of heart valves [29], polycaprolactone and gelatin nanocomposites [40] and poly(glycerol sebacate) reinforced with Bioglass [41] for cardiac patches.

MICELLES

Micelles are amphiphilic delivery systems composed of either polymer or lipids. The core of the micelles is lipophilic, whereas the outer shell is hydrophilic, which means that it can be used for the delivery of lipid-soluble drugs. The size of the micelle structure is usually between 10-100 nm and is formed spontaneously when the concentration of the surfactant surpasses the critical micelle concentration; more precisely, the free energy of the system is abridged. The micelle delivery system increases the bioavailability of the drug as it prolongs the circulation time owing to its hydrophilic shell and nanosize. Polymeric micelles are more favoured due to better stability, minimal toxicity, better drug loading and stability [42]. Furthermore, functionalization of the micelle surface is possible for targeted delivery additively, providing sustained and prolonged release of the drug. Stimuli-responsive micelles or ligand-based micelles can be explored for targeted delivery. External factors such as pH, light, temperature or enzymes have been exploited for delivery to vascular tissues. Additionally, nanosize favours better accumulation in the cardiac tissues, which renders them applicable in the treatment of CVDs [43].

DENDRIMERS

The term dendrimers has been coined from the Greek word 'dendron', meaning tree which suggests a structure with branches mimicking a tree. It has a 3-D structure with various functional groups on the surface, which makes it ideal for drug delivery and diagnosis. They have the ability to provide controlled/sustained delivery, prolong half-life, reduced toxicity and improved bioavailability. The most promising application is its ability to serve as a platform for functionalization [44]. However, the high quantity of branches on their exterior makes them highly cationic or anionic, which can cause toxicity [45]. Much effort has been put to eliminate the toxicity hazard of dendrimers by modifying the central core.

NANOTECHNOLOGY IN DIAGNOSTIC IMAGING

The diagnosis of disease usually involves the detection of molecular and cellular level functionalities. This is possible with the help of nanoprobes which offers good contrast [46], prolonged systemic circulation [47], high payload [48] and the ability to incorporate multiple contrast agents [49]. Quantum dots provide good fluorescence with high efficiency and particularly useful for imaging thick tissues. One of the researchers has used micellar-coated quantum dot core nanoparticles for the imaging of macrophages in atherosclerosis [50]. Some authors have established that perfluorocarbon-based microemulsions can be used as contrast agents to target $\alpha_v\beta_3$-integrin [51], fibrin [52] or collagen III [53], which play predominant roles in atherosclerotic plaque formation. Iron oxide nanoparticles, particularly super-paramagnetic iron oxide nanoparticles (SPIONS) are most commonly used as MRI contrast agents because of biocompatibility [54]. The nanoparticles comprising metals that serve as CT contrast agents are iodine, bismuth and gold. Furthermore, various ligands such as sugars, proteins, peptides, antibody fragments, antibodies and aptamers can be anchored to the delivery system to facilitate active targeting to the desired imaging site. The size of the delivery system cannot be overlooked as it attends a prominent part in targeting. During the course of a cardiovascular complication often the tissues are inflamed which possess highly permeable vasculature. The delivery of the formulation will be easy if the size is small. However, reducing the size of the contrast agent can be challenging as it may affect their contrast [55]. For example, the emission wavelength of quantum dots reduces on decreasing the size. Therefore, a proper balance between the size of the contrast agent and tuning the contrast should be decided. Some of the nanocarriers that are used for the management of diagnostics of CVDs are discussed (Table **1**).

Table 1. Some nanotechnological formulation for treatment of cardiovascular diseases for diagnostic applications.

Types of Nanoparticles	Relevant Features	References
Iron oxide- PLGA nanoparticles	Early detection of a thrombus and in the dynamic monitoring of the thrombolytic efficiency using MRI.	[56]
Platelet microparticle (PMP)-inspired nanovesicles	Targeting to GP IIb/IIIa and P-selectin achieved and demonstrated delayed thrombus growth	[57]
Urokinase functionalize magnetic nanoparticles	Promoted dissolution of thrombus	[58]

(Table 1) cont.....

Types of Nanoparticles	Relevant Features	References
Nattokinase loaded polyethylene glycol-polyglutamic acid peptide dendrimers	Good thrombolytic activity and improved the viability of macrophage cells	[59]
Manganese and G8 dendrimers targeted to oxidation-specific epitopes and functionalized with antibody MDA2	Potential as imaging agent of *in vivo* detection of macrophage-rich plaques of atherosclerotic lesions	[60]
Nano-fibrinolytic agent (CLIO-FXIII-PEG-tPA) crosslinked dextran-coated iron oxide nanoparticle	Detection of macrophages with phagocytic activity and cathepsin activity in transplant graft rejection.	[61]
Thrombin-activatable fluorescent peptide (TAP) incorporated silica-coated gold nanoparticles	Useful for direct thrombus imaging and therapy	[62]

CONCLUSION

Until recently, it was believed that nanotechnology could only serve as a therapeutic tool to alienate the pharmaceutical and pharmacological constraints of cardiovascular drugs. However, research in the area of diagnostic imaging has proved otherwise. CVD has become an economic burden as it is the first stage in the progression of more complex diseases such as diabetes. It impacts people's lives as it is the foremost cause of morbidity and death. Revolution in genetics, molecular and cellular biology makes nanotechnology one of the sought-after approaches to bridge the gap between treatment and diagnosis. A combination of these, known as theranostics, is the technology of the era that will help clinicians to achieve their objectives. Nonetheless, in spite of much progress, limitations of nanotechnology such as toxicity, stability, poor targeting efficiency and difficulty in scaling-up makes it challenging for designing a successful formulation. Further, much of the efficacy studies were carried out *in-vivo* on animal models; therefore, its suitability in humans cannot be ruled out. Therefore, studies in future should be focussed on formulating such a delivery system which will help in combatting the technological challenges and make nanotechnology a successful strategy for the treatment and diagnosis of CVDs.

CONSENT FOR PUBLICATION

Not Applicable.

CONFLICT OF INTEREST

The author confirms that this chapter contents have no conflict of interest.

ACKNOWLEDGEMENT

Declared none.

REFERENCES

[1]   https://www.who.int/news-room/fact-sheets/detail/cardiovascular-diseases-(cvds)

[2]   Weaver J. Insights into how calcium forms plaques in arteries pave the way for new treatments for heart disease. PLoS Biol 2013; 11(4)e1001533
[http://dx.doi.org/10.1371/journal.pbio.1001533] [PMID: 23585734]

[3]   Banach M, Serban C, Sahebkar A, *et al.* Impact of statin therapy on coronary plaque composition: a systematic review and meta-analysis of virtual histology intravascular ultrasound studies. BMC Med 2015; 13: 229.
[http://dx.doi.org/10.1186/s12916-015-0459-4] [PMID: 26385210]

[4]   Gupta AK, Gupta M. Synthesis and surface engineering of iron oxide nanoparticles for biomedical applications. Biomaterials 2005; 26(18): 3995-4021.
[http://dx.doi.org/10.1016/j.biomaterials.2004.10.012] [PMID: 15626447]

[5]   Patel DN, Bailey SR. Nanotechnology in cardiovascular medicine. Catheter Cardiovasc Interv 2007; 69(5): 643-54.
[http://dx.doi.org/10.1002/ccd.21060] [PMID: 17390307]

[6]   De Jong WH, Borm PJA. Drug delivery and nanoparticles:applications and hazards. Int J Nanomedicine 2008; 3(2): 133-49.
[http://dx.doi.org/10.2147/IJN.S596] [PMID: 18686775]

[7]   Akbarzadeh A, Rezaei-Sadabady R, Davaran S, *et al.* Liposome: classification, preparation, and applications. Nanoscale Res Lett 2013; 8(1): 102.
[http://dx.doi.org/10.1186/1556-276X-8-102] [PMID: 23432972]

[8]   Sahoo SK, Labhasetwar V. Nanotech approaches to drug delivery and imaging. Drug Discov Today 2003; 8(24): 1112-20.
[http://dx.doi.org/10.1016/S1359-6446(03)02903-9] [PMID: 14678737]

[9]   Meng QH, Jamal W, Hart SL, McEwan JR. Application to vascular adventitia of a nonviral vector for TIMP-1 gene therapy to prevent intimal hyperplasia. Hum Gene Ther 2006; 17(7): 717-27.
[http://dx.doi.org/10.1089/hum.2006.17.717] [PMID: 16839271]

[10]   Pfosser A, Thalgott M, Büttner K, *et al.* Liposomal Hsp90 cDNA induces neovascularization *via* nitric oxide in chronic ischemia. Cardiovasc Res 2005; 65(3): 728-36.
[http://dx.doi.org/10.1016/j.cardiores.2004.10.019] [PMID: 15664400]

[11]   Kaneda Y, Saeki Y, Morishita R. Gene therapy using HVJ-liposomes: the best of both worlds? Mol Med Today 1999; 5(7): 298-303.
[http://dx.doi.org/10.1016/S1357-4310(99)01482-3] [PMID: 10377521]

[12]   Immordino ML, Dosio F, Cattel L. Stealth liposomes: review of the basic science, rationale, and clinical applications, existing and potential. Int J Nanomedicine 2006; 1(3): 297-315.
[PMID: 17717971]

[13]   Levchenko TS, Hartner WC, Torchilin VP. Liposomes in diagnosis and treatment of cardiovascular disorders. Methodist DeBakey Cardiovasc J 2012; 8(1): 36-41.
[http://dx.doi.org/10.14797/mdcj-8-1-36] [PMID: 22891109]

[14]   Zhang N, Li C, Zhou D, *et al.* Cyclic RGD functionalized liposomes encapsulating urokinase for thrombolysis. Acta Biomater 2018; 70: 227-36.
[http://dx.doi.org/10.1016/j.actbio.2018.01.038] [PMID: 29412186]

[15]   Das M, Das DK. Lipid raft in cardiac health and disease. Curr Cardiol Rev 2009; 5(2): 105-11.
[http://dx.doi.org/10.2174/157340309788166660] [PMID: 20436850]

[16]   Bendas G, Krause A, Schmidt R, Vogel J, Rothe U. Selectins as new targets for immunoliposome-mediated drug delivery. A potential way of anti-inflammatory therapy. Pharm Acta Helv 1998; 73(1): 19-26.

[http://dx.doi.org/10.1016/S0031-6865(97)00043-5] [PMID: 9708035]

[17]   Gunawan RC, Auguste DT. Immunoliposomes that target endothelium *in vitro* are dependent on lipid raft formation. Mol Pharm 2010; 7(5): 1569-75.
[http://dx.doi.org/10.1021/mp9003095] [PMID: 20666515]

[18]   Tekabe Y, Einstein AJ, Johnson LL, Khaw BA. Targeting very small model lesions pretargeted with bispecific antibody with 99mTc-labeled high-specific radioactivity polymers. Nucl Med Commun 2010; 31(4): 320-7.
[http://dx.doi.org/10.1097/MNM.0b013e32833576e8] [PMID: 20087237]

[19]   Erdoğan S, Ozer AY, Volkan B, Caner B, Bilgili H. Thrombus localization by using streptokinase containing vesicular systems. Drug Deliv 2006; 13(4): 303-9.
[http://dx.doi.org/10.1080/10717540600559544] [PMID: 16766472]

[20]   Erdoğan S, Ozer AY, Bilgili H. *In vivo* behaviour of vesicular urokinase. Int J Pharm 2005; 295(1-2): 1-6.
[http://dx.doi.org/10.1016/j.ijpharm.2005.01.021] [PMID: 15847986]

[21]   Danila D, Partha R, Elrod DB, Lackey M, Casscells SW, Conyers JL. Antibody-labeled liposomes for CT imaging of atherosclerotic plaques: *in vitro* investigation of an anti-ICAM antibody-labeled liposome containing iohexol for molecular imaging of atherosclerotic plaques *via* computed tomography. Tex Heart Inst J 2009; 36(5): 393-403.
[PMID: 19876414]

[22]   Mulder WJM, Strijkers GJ, Griffioen AW, et al. A liposomal system for contrast-enhanced magnetic resonance imaging of molecular targets. Bioconjug Chem 2004; 15(4): 799-806.
[http://dx.doi.org/10.1021/bc049949r] [PMID: 15264867]

[23]   Almer G, Wernig K, Saba-Lepek M, et al. Adiponectin-coated nanoparticles for enhanced imaging of atherosclerotic plaques. Int J Nanomedicine 2011; 6: 1279-90.
[PMID: 21753879]

[24]   Pont I, Calatayud-Pascual A, López-Castellano A, et al. Anti-angiogenic drug loaded liposomes: Nanotherapy for early atherosclerotic lesions in mice 2018; 13(1): e0190540.

[25]   Cipriano AF, De Howitt N, Gott SC, Miller C, Rao MP, Liu H. Bone marrow stromal cell adhesion and morphology on micro- and sub-micropatterned titanium. J Biomed Nanotechnol 2014; 10(4): 660-8.
[http://dx.doi.org/10.1166/jbn.2014.1760] [PMID: 24734518]

[26]   Nahrendorf M, Zhang H, Hembrador S, et al. Nanoparticle PET-CT imaging of macrophages in inflammatory atherosclerosis. Circulation 2008; 117(3): 379-87.
[http://dx.doi.org/10.1161/CIRCULATIONAHA.107.741181] [PMID: 18158358]

[27]   Kanno S, Wu YJ, Lee PC, et al. Macrophage accumulation associated with rat cardiac allograft rejection detected by magnetic resonance imaging with ultrasmall superparamagnetic iron oxide particles. Circulation 2001; 104(8): 934-8.
[http://dx.doi.org/10.1161/hc3401.093148] [PMID: 11514382]

[28]   McCarthy JR, Sazonova IY, Erdem SS, et al. Multifunctional nanoagent for thrombus-targeted fibrinolytic therapy. Nanomedicine (Lond) 2012; 7(7): 1017-28.
[http://dx.doi.org/10.2217/nnm.11.179] [PMID: 22348271]

[29]   Kidane AG, Burriesci G, Edirisinghe M, Ghanbari H, Bonhoeffer P, Seifalian AM. A novel nanocomposite polymer for development of synthetic heart valve leaflets. Acta Biomater 2009; 5(7): 2409-17.
[http://dx.doi.org/10.1016/j.actbio.2009.02.025] [PMID: 19497802]

[30]   Thapa A, Webster TJ, Haberstroh KM. Polymers with nano-dimensional surface features enhance bladder smooth muscle cell adhesion. J Biomed Mater Res A 2003; 67(4): 1374-83.
[http://dx.doi.org/10.1002/jbm.a.20037] [PMID: 14624525]

[31]   Luo FHeyderman L. Solak H,Thomson T, Best M. Nanoscale perpendicular magnetic island arrays fabricated by extreme ultraviolet interference lithography. Appl Phys Lett 2008; 92(10)102505
[http://dx.doi.org/10.1063/1.2841821]

[32]   Suh KY, Lee HH. Capillary force lithography: large-area patterning, selforganization, and anisotropic dewetting. Adv Funct Mater 2002; 12(6-7): 405-13.
[http://dx.doi.org/10.1002/1616-3028(20020618)12:6/7<405::AID-ADFM405>3.0.CO;2-1]

[33]   Hon K, Li L, Hutchings I. Direct writing technologydadvances and developments. CIRP Annal Manuf Technol 2008; 57(2): 601-20.
[http://dx.doi.org/10.1016/j.cirp.2008.09.006]

[34]   Cipriano AF, Miller C, Liu H. Anodic growth and biomedical applications of TiO2 nanotubes. J Biomed Nanotechnol 2014; 10(10): 2977-3003.
[http://dx.doi.org/10.1166/jbn.2014.1927] [PMID: 25992426]

[35]   Wetteland CL, Nguyen NY, Liu H. Concentration-dependent behaviors of bone marrow derived mesenchymal stem cells and infectious bacteria toward magnesium oxide nanoparticles. Acta Biomater 2016; 35: 341-56.
[http://dx.doi.org/10.1016/j.actbio.2016.02.032] [PMID: 26923529]

[36]   Qi C, Zhu YJ, Lu BQ, *et al.* Hydroxyapatite hierarchically nanostructured porous hollow microspheres: rapid, sustainable microwave-hydrothermal synthesis by using creatine phosphate as an organic phosphorus source and application in drug delivery and protein adsorption. Chemistry 2013; 19(17): 5332-41.
[http://dx.doi.org/10.1002/chem.201203886] [PMID: 23460360]

[37]   Ignarro LJ. Nitric oxide: a unique endogenous signaling molecule in vascular biology (Nobel lecture). Angew Chem Int Ed 1999; 38(13-14): 1882-92.
[http://dx.doi.org/10.1002/(SICI)1521-3773(19990712)38:13/14<1882::AID-ANIE1882>3.0.CO;2-V]

[38]   Medley CD, Smith JE, Tang Z, Wu Y, Bamrungsap S, Tan W. Gold nanoparticle-based colorimetric assay for the direct detection of cancerous cells. Anal Chem 2008; 80(4): 1067-72.
[http://dx.doi.org/10.1021/ac702037y] [PMID: 18198894]

[39]   Al Meslmani BMMG, Mahmoud GF, Bakowsky U. Development of expanded polytetrafluoroethylene cardiovascular graft platform based on immobilization of poly lactic-co-glycolic acid nanoparticles using a wet chemical modification technique. Int J Pharm 2017; 529(1-2): 238-44.
[http://dx.doi.org/10.1016/j.ijpharm.2017.06.091] [PMID: 28689963]

[40]   Shevach M, Maoz BM, Feiner R, Shapira A, Dvir T. Nanoengineering gold particle composite fibers for cardiac tissue engineering. J Mater Chem B 1 2013; 39: 5210-7.

[41]   Chen Q, Jin L, Cook WD, Mohn D, Lagerqvist EL, Elliott DA, *et al.* Elastomeric nanocomposites as cell delivery vehicles and cardiac support devices. Soft Matter 2010; 6(19): 4715-26.
[http://dx.doi.org/10.1039/c0sm00213e]

[42]   Rösler A, Vandermeulen GW, Klok H-A. Advanced drug delivery devices *via* self-assembly of amphiphilic block copolymers. Adv Drug Deliv Rev 2012; 64: 270-9.
[http://dx.doi.org/10.1016/j.addr.2012.09.026] [PMID: 11733119]

[43]   Musacchio T, Torchilin VP. Advances in polymeric and lipid-core micelles as drug delivery systems. 2013.
[http://dx.doi.org/10.1201/b13758-4]

[44]   Abbasi E, Aval SF, Akbarzadeh A, *et al.* Dendrimers: synthesis, applications, and properties. Nanoscale Res Lett 2014; 9(1): 247.
[http://dx.doi.org/10.1186/1556-276X-9-247] [PMID: 24994950]

[45]   Janaszewska A, Lazniewska J, Trzepiński P, Marcinkowska M, Klajnert-Maculewicz B. Cytotoxicity of Dendrimers. Biomolecules 2019; 9(8): 1-23.
[http://dx.doi.org/10.3390/biom9080330] [PMID: 31374911]

[46]   Medintz IL, Uyeda HT, Goldman ER, Mattoussi H. Quantum dot bioconjugates for imaging, labelling and sensing. Nat Mater 2005; 4(6): 435-46.
[http://dx.doi.org/10.1038/nmat1390] [PMID: 15928695]

[47]   Klibanov AL, Maruyama K, Torchilin VP, Huang L. Amphipathic polyethyleneglycols effectively prolong the circulation time of liposomes. FEBS Lett 1990; 268(1): 235-7.
[http://dx.doi.org/10.1016/0014-5793(90)81016-H] [PMID: 2384160]

[48]   Schmieder AH, Winter PM, Caruthers SD, *et al.* Molecular MR imaging of melanoma angiogenesis with alphanubeta3-targeted paramagnetic nanoparticles. Magn Reson Med 2005; 53(3): 621-7.
[http://dx.doi.org/10.1002/mrm.20391] [PMID: 15723405]

[49]   Nahrendorf M, Jaffer FA, Kelly KA, *et al.* Noninvasive vascular cell adhesion molecule-1 imaging identifies inflammatory activation of cells in atherosclerosis. Circulation 2006; 114(14): 1504-11.
[http://dx.doi.org/10.1161/CIRCULATIONAHA.106.646380] [PMID: 17000904]

[50]   Mulder WJM, Strijkers GJ, Briley-Saboe KC, *et al.* Molecular imaging of macrophages in atherosclerotic plaques using bimodal PEG-micelles. Magn Reson Med 2007; 58(6): 1164-70.
[http://dx.doi.org/10.1002/mrm.21315] [PMID: 18046703]

[51]   Winter PMCS, Caruthers SD, Zhang H, Williams TA, Wickline SA, Lanza GM. Antiangiogenic synergism of integrin-targeted fumagillin nanoparticles and atorvastatin in atherosclerosis. JACC Cardiovasc Imaging 2008; 1(5): 624-34.
[http://dx.doi.org/10.1016/j.jcmg.2008.06.003] [PMID: 19356492]

[52]   Winter PM, Cai K, Chen J, *et al.* Targeted PARACEST nanoparticle contrast agent for the detection of fibrin. Magn Reson Med 2006; 56(6): 1384-8.
[http://dx.doi.org/10.1002/mrm.21093] [PMID: 17089356]

[53]   Cyrus T, Abendschein DR, Caruthers SD, *et al.* MR three-dimensional molecular imaging of intramural biomarkers with targeted nanoparticles. J Cardiovasc Magn Reson 2006; 8(3): 535-41.
[http://dx.doi.org/10.1080/10976640600580296] [PMID: 16755843]

[54]   Corot C, Robert P, Idée J-M, Port M. Recent advances in iron oxide nanocrystal technology for medical imaging. Adv Drug Deliv Rev 2006; 58(14): 1471-504.
[http://dx.doi.org/10.1016/j.addr.2006.09.013] [PMID: 17116343]

[55]   Cormode DP, Skajaa T, Fayad ZA, Mulder WJM. Nanotechnology in medical imaging: probe design and applications. Arterioscler Thromb Vasc Biol 2009; 29(7): 992-1000.
[http://dx.doi.org/10.1161/ATVBAHA.108.165506] [PMID: 19057023]

[56]   Zhou J, Guo D, Zhang Y, Wu W, Ran H, Wang Z. Construction and evaluation of Fe_3O_4-based PLGA nanoparticles carrying rtPA used in the detection of thrombosis and in targeted thrombolysis. ACS Appl Mater Interfaces 2014; 6(8): 5566-76.
[http://dx.doi.org/10.1021/am406008k] [PMID: 24693875]

[57]   Pawlowski CL, Li W, Sun M, *et al.* Platelet microparticle-inspired clot-responsive nanomedicine for targeted fibrinolysis. Biomaterials 2017; 128(28): 94-108.
[http://dx.doi.org/10.1016/j.biomaterials.2017.03.012] [PMID: 28314136]

[58]   Bi F, Zhang J, Su Y, Tang YC, Liu JN. Chemical conjugation of urokinase to magnetic nanoparticles for targeted thrombolysis 2009.
[http://dx.doi.org/10.1016/j.biomaterials.2009.06.006]

[59]   Zhang SF, Lü S, Gao C, *et al.* Multiarm-polyethylene glycol-polyglutamic acid peptide dendrimer: Design, synthesis, and dissolving thrombus. J Biomed Mater Res A 2018; 106(6): 1687-96.
[http://dx.doi.org/10.1002/jbm.a.36375] [PMID: 29468794]

[60]   Nguyen TH, Bryant H, Shapsa A, *et al.* Manganese G8 dendrimers targeted to oxidation-specific epitopes: *in vivo* MR imaging of atherosclerosis. J Magn Reson Imaging 2015; 41(3): 797-805.
[http://dx.doi.org/10.1002/jmri.24606] [PMID: 24610640]

[61]   McCarthy JR, Sazonova IY, Erdem SS, *et al.* Multifunctional nanoagent for thrombus-targeted fibrinolytic therapy. Nanomedicine (Lond) 2012; 7(7): 1017-28.
[http://dx.doi.org/10.2217/nnm.11.179] [PMID: 22348271]

[62]   Kwon SP, Jeon S, Lee SH, *et al.* Thrombin-activatable fluorescent peptide incorporated gold nanoparticles for dual optical/computed tomography thrombus imaging. Biomaterials 2018; 150: 125-36.
[http://dx.doi.org/10.1016/j.biomaterials.2017.10.017] [PMID: 29035738]

CHAPTER 4

Nanotechnology-Based Molecular Imaging in Cardiovascular Disease

Fahima Dilnawaz[1,*] and Zeenat Iqbal[2]

[1] *Laboratory of Nanomedicine, Institute of Life Sciences, Nalco Square, Chandrasekharpur, Bhubaneswar-751023, Odisha, India*

[2] *Nanomedicine Laboratory, Department of Pharmaceutics, School of Pharmaceutical Education & Research, Jamia Hamdard, New Delhi-110062, India*

Abstract: Nanoparticulate formulations have been valuable imaging tools in preclinical cardiovascular disease research. Nanocarriers' distinct properties are useful to carry out imaging with significant functional versatility, which is not achieved by traditional small-molecule agents. Various cardiovascular diseases (CVDs) require molecular and cellular mechanisms understanding, which will provide valuable insight towards theranostic (diagnostic and therapeutic) applications. Nanocarriers and radiolabeled nanoparticulate probes demonstrate their utility in several CVDs applications such as blood pool imaging and molecular imaging of ischemia, angiogenesis, atherosclerosis, and inflammation. Further, these emergent technologies need to address safety, toxicity and regulatory obligations for their clinical translation.

Keywords: Microbubble, Nanoparticles. Imaging, Quantum dots.

INTRODUCTION

Recently emphasis has been driven towards the primary or secondary prevention mode of treatment of cardiovascular disease. Consequent improvement of human health would lead to a quality life. Shifting towards the prevention of disease invites new challenges for translational research and stimulates the technological revolution of existing diagnostic procedures. For an easy and accurate diagnosis and therapy, molecular imaging plays a crucial role and has evolved as a fast-growing research field. Through this approach, vital information of physiologic, anatomic and molecular aspects of the disease can be obtained [1]. Currently, nanoparticle-based formulations have garnered enormous attention for the application of cardiovascular imaging and therapeutic delivery due to their better pharmacokinetic and biodistribution performance than that of small molecules [1].

---

* **Corresponding author Dr Fahima Dilnawaz:** Laboratory of Nanomedicine, Institute of Life Sciences, Nalco Square, Bhubanwswar-751023, Odisha, India. Tel: +91-674–2304341, 2304283, Fax: 91-674-2300728, E-mail: fahimadilnawaz@gmail.com

Outstandingly, nanoparticulate imaging agents are very helpful in signal amplification; these agents can be functionalized with functional entities such as targeting ligands for precise specificity. Imaging platform with the aid of nanoparticulate agents plays a significant role in imaging clots, thrombus, apoptosis-linked gene expression *etc*, which can be visualized by tracking. In imaging, the prime application is to image clogged blood vessels, defective valves, damaged heart muscles, *etc*. Till now, nanoparticle-based imaging agents have achieved inadequate clinical access as they require additional developmental features to overcome various functional limitations and related safety concerns. Further nanoparticles display the capability of cellular guidance in certain cardiovascular applications (Fig. **1**).

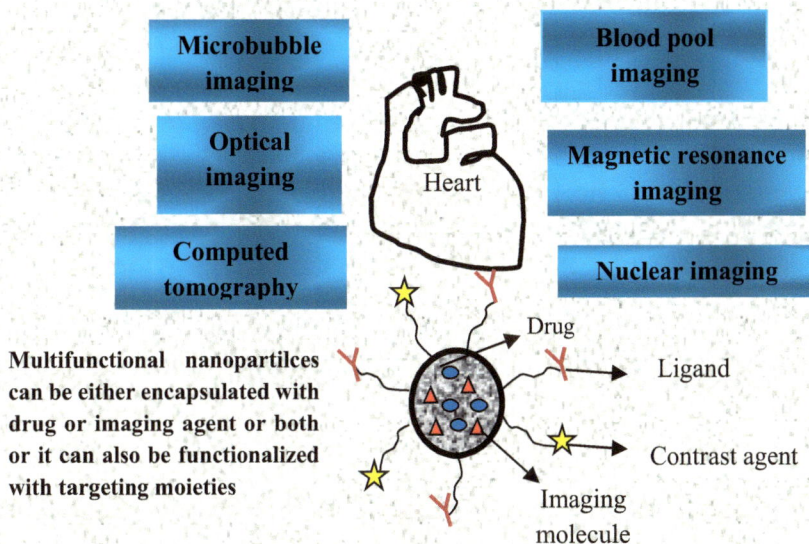

Fig. (1). Usage of multifunctional nanoparticles for various molecular imaging facility.

Nanoparticle-based cardiovascular imaging through Computed Tomography (CT), Magnetic Resonance Imaging (MRI), Positron Emission Tomography (PET) and Single Photon Emission Computed Tomography (SPECT) and its radiolabeled nanoparticulate probes have illustrated preclinical applications in blood pool imaging and molecular imaging of ischemia, angiogenesis, atherosclerosis, and inflammation [2 - 4]. In this chapter, various imaging modalities mediated through nanoparticles are discussed.

MICROBUBBLE BASED IMAGING

Microbubbles are the small gaseous particles between 1 and 10 μm, that are scattered with ultrasound waves giving enhanced contrast to the image during an echocardiogram [5]. An echocardiogram is a sonographic based imaging technique, which is an exquisite tool for the non-invasive and real-time diagnosis of physiological tissues and requires contrast agents for providing backscatter of sound waves to scanner head, which are usually gas-filled microbubbles (1-5μm in diameter) that are re-stabilized either with lipid, protein, polymers, or a mixture of these [6, 7]. Looking at the potentiality, researchers have engineered microbubbles to enable drug loading, improve circulation time, increase stability as well as molecular targeting [8]. Recently to provide multifunctionality, nanoparticles and microbubbles are complexed together. This complexion stabilizes the bubbles by modifying the interfacial tension and diffusivity of a gas bubble in liquid [9]. In an attempt, Dixon *et al.*, conjugated gold nanorods onto the lipid shell of the microbubbles through the gold–thiol linkage under the presence of the (pyridyldithio)propionyl group for *in vivo* photoacoustic imaging [10]. Ke *et al.*, complexed quantum dots and microbubbles *via* the electrostatic layer-by-layer technique that responded to the medical ultrasound to act as a contrast-enhanced agent [11]. In another study, Yang *et al.*, developed dual contrast agents of magnetic resonance and ultrasound imaging by embedding superparamagnetic iron oxide nanoparticle-microbubbles for imaging [12]. Molecular imaging is of paramount importance as it provides access to the identification of specific cell-surface tissue functionality receptors with targeted contrast agents. Lanza *et al.*, used a ligand-targeted acoustic nanoparticle system to identify the angioplasty-induced expression of tissue factor by smooth muscle cells within the tunica media. The result illustrated that the nanoemulsion was able to infiltrate into arterial walls after balloon injury and localize the expression of overstretch-induced tissue factor within pig carotid arteries proving to be a prognostically important predictor of subsequent restenosis [13]. Hamilton *et al.*, developed targeted echogenic immunoliposomes (ELIPs) for enhancement of intravascular ultrasound imaging of atherosclerosis. By functionalizing with anti-ICAM, anti-fibrinogen, anti-fibrin, and anti-VCAM antibodies (Ab/Abs), early and later atheroma components can be targeted by imaging [14]. Tiukinhoy-Laing *et al.*, entrapped tissue-plasminogen activator (tPA) for fibrin-targeted, ultrasound-directed and enhanced local delivery of a thrombolytic agent. After administration of tPA–ELIP the clot images are highlighted when compared to control [15]. VEGF peptides have angiogenic potential and resulted in therapeutic effectiveness. Hwang *et al.*, developed chitosan hydrogel nanoparticles loaded with vascular endothelial growth factor (VEGF) for the treatment of myocardial ischemia. Administration of chitosan peptides reduced the intensity of perfusion defects and increased vascular density as compared to control [16].

Optical Imaging: It is a non-invasive technique that uses light to probe cellular and molecular function in the living body. The most fruitful nanotechnology based optical agents are Quantum Dots (QDs) which can be used as fluorescent markers for diagnostic purposes. They have unique fluorescent properties, which make them useful as probes for both *in-vitro* and *in-vivo* imaging [2]. The basis of optical imaging is that the transmission window of biological tissues falls within the near-infrared region (NIR) (650-800nm) and investigation within this range allows for deeper light penetration and reduced light scattering, thus producing increased image contrast with an excellent sensitivity of detection [2, 17]. Stem cells show promise for the repair of damaged cardiac tissue. Traditional tracking agents such as fluorescent dyes fail to illuminate delivered cells effectively in the heart. In this regard, Rosen *et al.*, developed quantum dot (QD) nanoparticles to label human mesenchymal stem cells for long-term tracking in rat hearts [18].

NANOPARTICLE MEDIATED COMPUTED TOMOGRAPHY

In the near future, nanoparticles can be used as a contrast agent for imaging atherosclerotic plaques in patients with coronary and peripheral vascular diseases non-invasively. Sudden fibrous cap disruption of 'high-risk' atherosclerotic plaques can trigger the formation of an occlusive thrombus in coronary arteries, causing acute coronary syndromes. For preventing ischemic events, early identification of high-risk plaques is a necessary step. The high-risk atherosclerotic plaques are characterized particularly with a high density of macrophages. In this regard, Hyafil *et al.*, developed and used iodinated nanoparticles and found that nanoparticles get accumulated in the macrophages within atherosclerotic plaques in rabbits for clinical evaluation of coronary arteries with CT [19]. Currently used iodinated contrast media in CT is associated with the risk of contrast induced nephropathy [20]. Several other elements having high atomic no. such as gold, bismuth, iron, have also been used, in which gold is found to be more useful as it gives high contrast differences, resistant to oxidation at physiological conditions as well as has plasmon resonance in the visible region (400-800 nm) [21]. Kim *et al.*, developed gold nanoparticles (GNPs) coated with polyethylene glycol (PEG) to impart antibiofouling properties, which extends their lifetime in the bloodstream. With administration into rats, the PEG-coated GNPs illustrated higher blood circulation time and showed clear demarcation of cardiac ventricles and great vessels in CT images [21].

NANOPARTICLES FOR MAGNETIC RESONANCE IMAGING

MRI has emerged as a novel tool for the diagnosis of several cardiovascular complications. It requires powerful magnetic fields and radiofrequency waves to generate images of internal structures. It uses metals having high magnetism (such as cobalt or iron) or decorated with paramagnetic or superparamagnetic elements like Gadolinium with carriers such as liposomes, dendrimers, perfluorocarbon nanoemulsions, micelles, *etc.* Basically, there are three MRI techniques which are off-resonance, T_1, T_2 [22]. An MRI contrast agent accelerates the rate of T_1 and T_2 relaxation. A paramagnetic contrast agent such as chelates of Gadolinium accelerates longitudinal T_1 relaxation and produces 'bright' contrast. Superparamagnetic agents such as Iron oxide nanoparticles primarily increase the rate of dephasing or transverse T_2 relaxation and produce 'dark' contrast, while Off resonance imaging generates positive contrast [4, 23]. Lanza *et al.*, reported the efficacy of perfluorocarbon nanoparticles for a broad spectrum asymptomatic atherosclerotic disease to acute myocardial infarction or stroke [24]. Winter *et al.*, demonstrated the potentiality of $\alpha_v\beta_3$–targeted fumagillin paramagnetic nanoparticles to quantify atherosclerotic angiogenesis. These targeted nanoparticles reduced the neovascular signa MR molecular imaging and demonstrated the acute antiangiogenic effects. When combined with atorvastatin, these nanoparticles could be prolonged representing a potential strategy to evaluate antiangiogenic treatment and plaque stability [25]. Amirbekian *et al.*, developed Gd-containing micelles, anti-CD36 immunomicelles and Fc-micelles, which can bind to human macrophages. These nanoparticles demonstrated improved MR detection in human aortic atherosclerosis [26]. Another approach for T_1 signal amplification is the use of dendrimers which utilize effective cellular internalization and concentration of agent to build signal. Martina *et al.*, developed PEGylated superparamagnetic liposomes to assess the efficiency as a contrast agent for MR. With the intravenous injection, the contrast agent provided the first direct evidence of the stealthiness of PEGylated magnetic-fluid-loaded liposomes in rats [27].

NANOPARTICLE-BASED NUCLEAR IMAGING

Nuclear imaging modalities like Positron Emission Tomography (PET) and Single Photon Emission Computed Tomography (SPECT) produce 3-D images of functional processes in the body, which are commonly used for the early diagnosis of various cardiac abnormalities [28]. The main difference between PET and SPECT is that SPECT emits gamma rays (by Tc-99m, Xe-133) while PET includes positron emitters (such as F-18, I-124), PET technique is more sensitive than SPECT technique. The ability to detect and quantify macrophage accumulation can provide important diagnostic and prognostic information for atherosclerotic plaque. van der Valk *et al.*, conducted the first clinical trial using prednisolone conjugated long-circulating liposomal nanoparticles in patients with atherosclerosis, which accumulated in macrophages upon intravenous administration. The *ex vivo* analysis demonstrated liposomal delivery to plaque macrophages, with no localized anti-inflammatory effects detected with ^{18}F-FDG PET/CT. Despite the lack of efficacy, this study demonstrates the clinical feasibility of nanomedicine delivery in the clinical management of the cardiovascular disease [29]. Seo *et al*., synthesized dendritic form of LyP-1 9 (a cyclic 9-amino acid peptide, binds to p32 proteins on activated macrophages) for imaging by conjugating imaging probes for optical and PET studies. For PET-CT studies, (LyP-1)$_4$- and (ARAL)$_4$-dendrimer-6-BAT were labeled with ^{64}Cu ($t_{1/2}$ = 12.7 h) and intravenously injected into the atherosclerotic (ApoE$^{-/-}$) mice. After two hours PET-CT coregistered images demonstrated greater uptake of the (LyP-1)$_4$-dendrimer-^{64}Cu than the (ARAL)$_4$-dendrimer-^{64}Cu in the aortic root and descending aorta [30]. Chemokine receptor 5 (CCR5) is an active participant in the late stage of atherosclerosis and is being used as a prognostic biomarker for plaque stability. Biocompatible poly(methyl methacrylate)-core/polyethylene glycol-shell amphiphilic comb-like nanoparticle was prepared with controlled conjugation and polymerization and labeled with ^{64}Cu for CCR5 imaging in the ApoE$^{-/-}$ wire-injury model. Post intravenous administration, improved blood signaling, radiolabeling specific activity, and elevated targeting efficiency of amphiphilic ^{64}Cu-DOTA-DAPTA-comb were observed compared to ^{64}Cu-DOTA-DAPTA peptide alone [3]. Emerging macrophage-targeting therapeutics provide better roles of macrophages in human disease while identifying the risk for complications. Keliher *et al*., developed carboxymethyl polyglucose polymers based nanoparticles called "macrin" that are considered glycogen biomimetics as they lack the central glycogenic core. For PET imaging macrins are modified with ^{18}F (termed Macroflor). Macroflor is enriched in cardiac and plaque macrophages, which in turn increases the PET signal in murine infarcts and rabbit atherosclerotic plaques, suggesting macroflor to be a clinical tool to non-invasively monitor macrophage biology [31]. Nuclear imaging techniques have been used for arteriosclerosis-associated inflammatory events, such as those described by Nahrendorf *et al*., He used epicholrohydrin-cross linked dextran-coated iron oxide nanoparticles for imaging of lesions *in-vivo* [32]. Similarly, Narula *et al*., used Annexin V, which was radio-labelled with Tc-99m for imaging of apoptosis in myocardial infarction as well as inflammation associated with it [33]. Chrastina *et al*., described the use of I-125 as a SPECT imaging agent for biodistribution of silver nanoparticles in mice [34].

NANOPARTICLES FOR BLOOD POOL IMAGING

Blood pool agents are, in other words, known as (intravascular contrast agents) having a large size and better relaxivity to prevent diffusion through vascular epithelium [35]. These blood pool contrast agents stay in circulation up to an hour, allowing available window time for imaging. In this regard, the designed nanoparticulate formulations are potentially useful as blood pool imaging agents as they can be extended for circulation with minimal extravasation into the surrounding tissue. Further, PEGylation of the nanoparticulate formulations provides long circulation times. Conventional small molecule contrast agent overestimates intramyocardial blood volume because of significant first-pass myocardial extraction [36]. Atherosclerosis, a chronic inflammatory vascular disease, leads to myocardial infarction and cerebrovascular events, in which the enlarged plaque lesions constrict the luminal surface of the artery and reduce the blood flow. In a study, Trivedi *et al.*, illustrated accumulation of FeO-NP in atherosclerotic plaques that are rich in macrophages when injected into patients with severe internal carotid artery stenosis. In MRI, the accumulation of FeO-NP leads to local reduction in T_2*-weighted signals and enhancement of MRI contrast [37]. Monocytes and macrophages invade the arterial intima to amplify local inflammation through the secretion of cytokines, reactive oxygen species, and proteolytic enzymes. Imaging of lesional monocytes and macrophages acts as a biomarker of disease progression. Majumdar *et al.*, utilized dextran nanoparticles labeled with desferoxamine to chelate the PET isotope zirconium-89 (^{89}Zr). The PET/MRI revealed the high uptake of (89)Zr-DNP in the aortic root of apolipoprotein E knockout (ApoE(-/-)) mice compared to wild-type controls [38].

CONCLUSION

Cardiovascular disease-related molecular imaging exemplifies a vital role in early and precise diagnosis and therapy as it offers detailed molecular, physiologic and anatomic information of diseases. Recently significant attention has been drawn towards nanoparticle-based approach due to the ease of synthesis, integration of multiple functional moieties, *etc*. In this regard application of nanotechnology-mediated formulation has eventually generated a theranostic revolution towards cardiovascular diseases. With the advance in the understanding of cardiovascular sciences, better designing approach of nanoparticles could yield better pathophysiological details of cardiovascular diseases that can be translated into the clinic.

CONSENT FOR PUBLICATION

Not Applicable.

CONFLICT OF INTEREST

The author confirms that this chapter contents have no conflict of interest.

ACKNOWLEDGEMENT

FD gratefully acknowledges Dept. of Science and Technology, Govt. of India, for the financial grant [SR/WOS-A/LS-448/2017(G)] in the form of women scientist fellowship (WOS-A).

REFERENCES

[1]   McCarthy JR. Nanomedicine and cardiovascular disease. Curr Cardiovasc Imaging Rep 2010; 3(1): 42-9.
        [http://dx.doi.org/10.1007/s12410-009-9002-3] [PMID: 20369034]

[2]   Dubertret B, Skourides P, Norris DJ, Noireaux V, Brivanlou AH, Libchaber A. *In vivo* imaging of quantum dots encapsulated in phospholipid micelles. Science 2002; 298(5599): 1759-62.
        [http://dx.doi.org/10.1126/science.1077194] [PMID: 12459582]

[3]   Luehmann HP, Pressly ED, Detering L, *et al.* PET/CT imaging of chemokine receptor CCR5 in vascular injury model using targeted nanoparticle. J Nucl Med 2014; 55(4): 629-34.
        [http://dx.doi.org/10.2967/jnumed.113.132001] [PMID: 24591489]

[4]   Sosnovik DE, Nahrendorf M, Weissleder R. Magnetic nanoparticles for MR imaging: agents, techniques and cardiovascular applications. Basic Res Cardiol 2008; 103(2): 122-30.
        [http://dx.doi.org/10.1007/s00395-008-0710-7] [PMID: 18324368]

[5]   Karamanou M, Papaioannou TG, Stefanadis C, Androutsos G. Genesis of ultrasonic microbubbles: a quick historical overview. Curr Pharm Des 2012; 18(15): 2115-7.
        [http://dx.doi.org/10.2174/138161212800099937] [PMID: 22352767]

[6]   Bokor D, Chambers JB, Rees PJ, Mant TG, Luzzani F, Spinazzi A. Clinical safety of SonoVue, a new contrast agent for ultrasound imaging, in healthy volunteers and in patients with chronic obstructive pulmonary disease. Invest Radiol 2001; 36(2): 104-9.
        [http://dx.doi.org/10.1097/00004424-200102000-00006] [PMID: 11224758]

[7]   Godin B, Sakamoto JH, Serda RE, Grattoni A, Bouamrani A, Ferrari M. Emerging applications of nanomedicine for the diagnosis and treatment of cardiovascular diseases. Trends Pharmacol Sci 2010; 31(5): 199-205.
        [http://dx.doi.org/10.1016/j.tips.2010.01.003] [PMID: 20172613]

[8]   Martin KH, Dayton PA. Current status and prospects for microbubbles in ultrasound theranostics. Wiley Interdiscip Rev Nanomed Nanobiotechnol 2013; 5(4): 329-45.
        [http://dx.doi.org/10.1002/wnan.1219] [PMID: 23504911]

[9]   Azmin M, Mohamedi G, Edirisinghe M, Stride EP. Dissolution of coated microbubbles: the effect of nanoparticles and surfactant concentration. Mater Sci Eng C 2012; 32(8): 2654-8.
        [http://dx.doi.org/10.1016/j.msec.2012.06.019]

[10]   Dixon AJ, Hu S, Klibanov AL, Hossack JA. Oscillatory dynamics and *in vivo* photoacoustic imaging performance of plasmonic nanoparticle-coated microbubbles. small 2015; 11(25): 3066-77.

[11]   Ke H, Xing Z, Zhao B, *et al.* Quantum-dot-modified microbubbles with bi-mode imaging capabilities. Nanotechnology 2009; 20(42)425105
        [http://dx.doi.org/10.1088/0957-4484/20/42/425105] [PMID: 19779227]

[12]   Yang F, Li Y, Chen Z, Zhang Y, Wu J, Gu N. Superparamagnetic iron oxide nanoparticle-embedded encapsulated microbubbles as dual contrast agents of magnetic resonance and ultrasound imaging. Biomaterials 2009; 30(23-24): 3882-90.
        [http://dx.doi.org/10.1016/j.biomaterials.2009.03.051] [PMID: 19395082]

[13]   Lanza GM, Abendschein DR, Hall CS, *et al. In vivo* molecular imaging of stretch-induced tissue factor in carotid arteries with ligand-targeted nanoparticles. J Am Soc Echocardiogr 2000; 13(6): 608-14.
        [http://dx.doi.org/10.1067/mje.2000.105840] [PMID: 10849515]

[14]   Hamilton AJ, Huang SL, Warnick D, *et al.* Intravascular ultrasound molecular imaging of atheroma components *in vivo*. J Am Coll Cardiol 2004; 43(3): 453-60.
        [http://dx.doi.org/10.1016/j.jacc.2003.07.048] [PMID: 15013130]

[15]   Tiukinhoy-Laing SD, Huang S, Klegerman M, Holland CK, McPherson DD. Ultrasound-facilitated thrombolysis using tissue-plasminogen activator-loaded echogenic liposomes. Thromb Res 2007; 119(6): 777-84.

[http://dx.doi.org/10.1016/j.thromres.2006.06.009] [PMID: 16887172]

[16]   Hwang H, Kwon J, Oh PS, Lee T-K, Na K-S, Lee C-M, *et al.* Peptide-loaded Nanoparticles ande Imaging for Individualized Treatment of Myocardial Ischemia. Radiology 2014; 273(1): 150-67.

[17]   Lidke DS, Nagy P, Heintzmann R, *et al.* Quantum dot ligands provide new insights into erbB/HER receptor-mediated signal transduction. Nat Biotechnol 2004; 22(2): 198-203.
        [http://dx.doi.org/10.1038/nbt929] [PMID: 14704683]

[18]   Rosen AB, Kelly DJ, Schuldt AJT, *et al.* Finding fluorescent needles in the cardiac haystack: tracking human mesenchymal stem cells labeled with quantum dots for quantitative *in vivo* three-dimensional fluorescence analysis. Stem Cells 2007; 25(8): 2128-38.
        [http://dx.doi.org/10.1634/stemcells.2006-0722] [PMID: 17495112]

[19]   Hyafil F, Cornily JC, Feig JE, *et al.* Noninvasive detection of macrophages using a nanoparticulate contrast agent for computed tomography. Nat Med 2007; 13(5): 636-41.
        [http://dx.doi.org/10.1038/nm1571] [PMID: 17417649]

[20]   Weisbord SD, Mor MK, Resnick AL, Hartwig KC, Palevsky PM, Fine MJ. Incidence and outcomes of contrast-induced AKI following computed tomography. Clin J Am Soc Nephrol 2008; 3(5): 1274-81.
        [http://dx.doi.org/10.2215/CJN.01260308] [PMID: 18463172]

[21]   Kim D, Park S, Lee JH, Jeong YY, Jon S. Antibiofouling polymer-coated gold nanoparticles as a contrast agent for *in vivo* X-ray computed tomography imaging. J Am Chem Soc 2007; 129(24): 7661-5.
        [http://dx.doi.org/10.1021/ja071471p] [PMID: 17530850]

[22]   Smith RC, McCarthy S. Physics of magnetic resonance. J Reprod Med 1992; 37(1): 19-26.
        [PMID: 1548634]

[23]   Cunningham CH, Arai T, Yang PC, McConnell MV, Pauly JM, Conolly SM. Positive contrast magnetic resonance imaging of cells labeled with magnetic nanoparticles. Magn Reson Med 2005; 53(5): 999-1005.
        [http://dx.doi.org/10.1002/mrm.20477] [PMID: 15844142]

[24]   Lanza GM, Winter PM, Caruthers SD, *et al.* Nanomedicine opportunities for cardiovascular disease with perfluorocarbon nanoparticles. Nanomedicine (Lond) 2006; 1(3): 321-9.
        [http://dx.doi.org/10.2217/17435889.1.3.321] [PMID: 17716162]

[25]   Winter PM, Neubauer AM, Caruthers SD, *et al.* Endothelial alpha(v)beta3 integrin-targeted fumagillin nanoparticles inhibit angiogenesis in atherosclerosis. Arterioscler Thromb Vasc Biol 2006; 26(9): 2103-9.
        [http://dx.doi.org/10.1161/01.ATV.0000235724.11299.76] [PMID: 16825592]

[26]   Amirbekian V, Lipinski MJ, Frias JC, Amirbekian S, Briley-Saebo KC, Mani V, *et al.* MR imaging of human atherosclerosis using immunomicelles molecularly targeted to macrophages 2009.
        [http://dx.doi.org/10.1186/1532-429X-11-S1-P83]

[27]   Martina MS, Nicolas V, Wilhelm C, Ménager C, Barratt G, Lesieur S. The *in vitro* kinetics of the interactions between PEG-ylated magnetic-fluid-loaded liposomes and macrophages. Biomaterials 2007; 28(28): 4143-53.
        [http://dx.doi.org/10.1016/j.biomaterials.2007.05.025] [PMID: 17574668]

[28]   Cormode DP, Skajaa T, Fayad ZA, Mulder WJM. Nanotechnology in medical imaging: probe design and applications. Arterioscler Thromb Vasc Biol 2009; 29(7): 992-1000.
        [http://dx.doi.org/10.1161/ATVBAHA.108.165506] [PMID: 19057023]

[29]   van der Valk FM, van Wijk DF, Lobatto ME, *et al.* Prednisolone-containing liposomes accumulate in human atherosclerotic macrophages upon intravenous administration. Nanomedicine (Lond) 2015; 11(5): 1039-46.
        [http://dx.doi.org/10.1016/j.nano.2015.02.021] [PMID: 25791806]

[30]   Seo JW, Baek H, Mahakian LM, *et al.* (64)Cu-labeled LyP-1-dendrimer for PET-CT imaging of

atherosclerotic plaque. Bioconjug Chem 2014; 25(2): 231-9.
[http://dx.doi.org/10.1021/bc400347s] [PMID: 24433095]

[31]   Keliher EJ, Ye YX, Wojtkiewicz GR, *et al.* Polyglucose nanoparticles with renal elimination and macrophage avidity facilitate PET imaging in ischaemic heart disease. Nat Commun 2017; 8: 14064.
[http://dx.doi.org/10.1038/ncomms14064] [PMID: 28091604]

[32]   Nahrendorf M, Jaffer FA, Kelly KA, *et al.* Noninvasive vascular cell adhesion molecule-1 imaging identifies inflammatory activation of cells in atherosclerosis. Circulation 2006; 114(14): 1504-11.
[http://dx.doi.org/10.1161/CIRCULATIONAHA.106.646380] [PMID: 17000904]

[33]   Narula J, Hofstra L. Imaging myocardial necrosis and apoptosis.Atlas of Nuclear cardiology Philadelphia: Current Medicine. 2003; pp. 197-216.
[http://dx.doi.org/10.1007/978-1-4615-6496-6_12]

[34]   Chrastina A, Schnitzer JE. Iodine-125 radiolabeling of silver nanoparticles for *in vivo* SPECT imaging. Int J Nanomedicine 2010; 5: 653-9.
[PMID: 20856841]

[35]   Chen HH, Josephson L, Sosnovik DE. Imaging of apoptosis in the heart with nanoparticle technology. Wiley Interdiscip Rev Nanomed Nanobiotechnol 2011; 3(1): 86-99.
[http://dx.doi.org/10.1002/wnan.115] [PMID: 20945336]

[36]   Canty JM Jr, Judd RM, Brody AS, Klocke FJ. First-pass entry of nonionic contrast agent into the myocardial extravascular space. Effects on radiographic estimates of transit time and blood volume. Circulation 1991; 84(5): 2071-8.
[http://dx.doi.org/10.1161/01.CIR.84.5.2071] [PMID: 1657448]

[37]   Trivedi RA, Mallawarachi C, U-King-Im JM, *et al.* Identifying inflamed carotid plaques using *in vivo* USPIO-enhanced MR imaging to label plaque macrophages. Arterioscler Thromb Vasc Biol 2006; 26(7): 1601-6.
[http://dx.doi.org/10.1161/01.ATV.0000222920.59760.df] [PMID: 16627809]

[38]   Majmudar MD, Yoo J, Keliher EJ, *et al.* Polymeric nanoparticle PET/MR imaging allows macrophage detection in atherosclerotic plaques. Circ Res 2013; 112(5): 755-61.
[http://dx.doi.org/10.1161/CIRCRESAHA.111.300576] [PMID: 23300273]

CHAPTER 5

Nanocarriers for Therapeutics Delivery of Cardiovascular Disease

Fahima Dilnawaz[1,*]

[1] *Laboratory of Nanomedicine, Institute of Life Sciences, Nalco Square, Chandrasekharpur, Bhubaneswar-751023, Odisha, India*

Abstract: Cardiovascular diseases are presently the leading cause of death worldwide. Prescribed drugs in terms of therapeutic modalities of clinical management have treated patients, but still a limitation exists. This administered drug displays unwanted health adversity due to the side effects. In this regard, the current focus has been drawn towards nanomedicine-based drug formulation, which illustrates better therapeutic ability, sustained release, bioavailability and less toxicity. To address this, various nanocarriers are developed and are being involved in and studied for clinical application. In this chapter, the potential application of different nanocarrier-based therapeutic delivery has been discussed.

Keywords: Coronary artery disease, Dendrimers, Liposomes, Nanomedicine, Polymeric.

INTRODUCTION

Cardiovascular diseases (CVDs) and administered medicine in the form of nanosize is called cardiac nanomedicine. With the advent of nanoformulation, the focus has been driven towards the establishment of innovative solutions to meet the challenge of current CVD treatments. Nanomedicine is the fastest emerging research area that can revolutionize the CVDs care system. The major emphasis of designing nanoformulation is to improve the pre-existing drugs' bioavailability, stability and safety. The nanoformulative drugs are continuously being improved to achieve protection from systemic degradation, to demonstrate reduced toxicity, immunogenicity, improved pharmacokinetics and increased half-life, bioavailability and precise biodistribution [1]. For targeted therapeutic application, these nanoparticles can be further functionalized with different classes of targeting moieties for selective delivery to the site of interest [2].

[*] **Corresponding author Dr Fahima Dilnawaz:** Laboratory of Nanomedicine, Institute of Life Sciences, Nalco Square, Bhubanwswar-751023, Odisha, India; +91-674 – 2304341, 2304283, Fax: 91-674-2300728, E-mail: fahimadilnawaz@gmail.com

Fahima Dilnawaz and Zeenat Iqbal (Eds.)

Various administrative routes, such as inhalation, oral administration, or intravenous injection, can be taken into account for CVDs. These nanocarriers can enter into the system through various strategies (Fig. **1**).

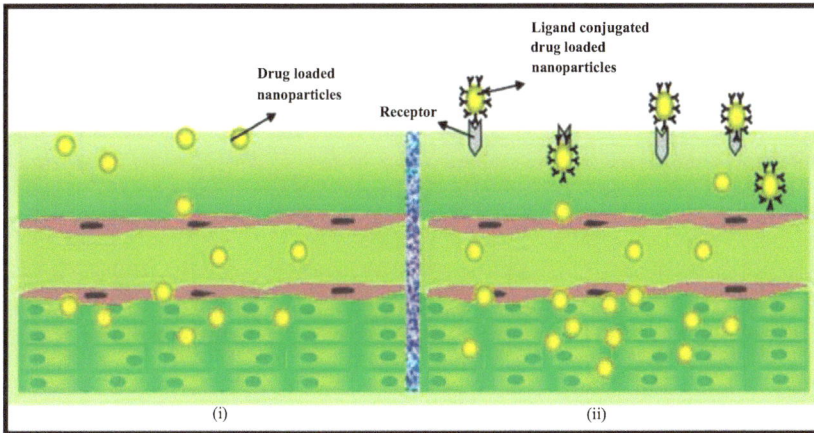

Fig. (1). (i) Passive targeting: In CVDs the chronic inflammatory process the increase of vascular permeability permits the drug loaded nanoparticles to pass through the blood vessels and reach the target site, **(ii)** Active targeting, the ligand conjugated nanoparticles are captured by the overexpressed receptors and are released at the site of action.

PASSIVE TARGETING

The passive targeting is diffusion mediated, as the microvascular endothelial cell space in normal tissue is dense and intact, but in the case of a tumor, the endothelial cells are richly vascularised, which has poor structural integrity and impaired lymphatic drainage system [3, 4]. In this case, the nanosized particles pass easily through the vascular wall and remain endocytosed in the tumor tissues, where they are largely accumulated due to the enhanced permeability and retention (EPR) effect [5]. The EPR effect is not only applicable to tumor tissues, but it can also be used in various CVD, such as the occurrence, and development of atherosclerosis (AS) is a chronic inflammatory process, where vascular permeability is often increased, which is very similar to that of solid tumors. The vascular endothelial permeability offers an effective means for the delivery of nanocarrier to deliver from the lumen side to the interior of the plaque. In another strategy, the nanocarriers can also enter the circulation and get ingested by the inflammatory cells (monocytes or macrophages) and further, these nanocarriers can migrate to plaque inflammation, allowing drugs to be delivered [6]. Additionally, for longer circulation in the blood-stream, the nanocarriers are PEGylated to decrease the immunogenicity, opsonization, and phagocytosis [7].

ACTIVE TARGETING

During the course of the development of CVDs, various vascular endothelial cells are in an inflammatory activation state, where certain molecules, such as intercellular cell adhesion molecule-1 (ICAM-1), vascular cell adhesion molecule-1 (VCAM-1), integrins, selectins, *etc.* are often overexpressed. These molecules can be functionalized with the nanocarriers for active targeting. These targeting moieties can bind effectively to the receptor sites of inflammation before they were taken up by endothelial cells [8]. Whether it is passive targeting or active targeting, the ultimate targeting efficiency is highly dependent upon the physicochemical properties (such as, particle size and distribution, targeting unit types, surface chemistry, morphology and density) of the nanoparticles [9]. Inside the body, different intrinsic biological factors (such as development stage, type as well as location of CVD and tumor, vascular wall shear rate, blood composition and its fluid type) also play an important role which greatly affects the targeting efficiency [10]. Moreover, the active targeting of the nanocarriers in clinical diagnosis and therapy is enormously attractive, but still, it faces great challenges because of the limitation of the discovery of an ideal target. Secondly, to combat many bottleneck problems of targeting, the formulation parameters need to be designed effectively.

NANOCARRIERS FOR THERAPEUTICS DELIVERY IN CVDS

Nanocarriers are the transport moiety, which is designed for drug loading and ligand functionalization. Most commonly used nanocarriers are micelles, polymeric, carbon-based materials, liposomes, dendrimers and other substances. Widely three types of nanoparticles (Fig. **2**) are used for cardiovascular study, which is being discussed below.

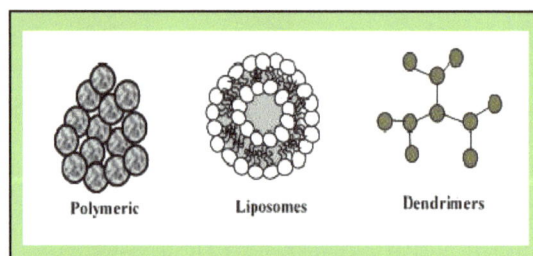

Fig. (2). Nanoparticles widely used for Cardiovascular disease.

POLYMERIC NANOMEDICINE

Ischaemic cardiac complication occurs when loss of blood supply to the tissue is lost, leading to cell death. With due course of time, the damage spreads, and the heart is unable to pump efficiently [11]. An increase in vascularisation to the affected area could reduce the symptoms of the patient. The angiogenic growth factor, vascular endothelial growth factor (VEGF), has been proposed to be useful for applications where the improved blood supply to the target tissue is required. A sustained release activity at the site of action is required to get the maximum benefit from VEGF therapy [12]. The sustained drug delivery at the site of action is often achieved by the delivery of therapeutic molecules in a particulate system. Nanoparticles are preferred for delivery to the areas that are in potential contact with the bloodstream, particularly for cardiac delivery, due to the reduced risk of embolization [13, 14]. In a particular study, O'Dwyer *et al.* complexed VEGF electrostatically with star -polyglutamic acid (PGA) polypeptides, which facilitated the sustained release activity upto 28 days. Further, the PGA-VEGF nanomedicines are loaded into hyaluronic acid hydrogel form a nano-in-gel system for a percutaneous delivery illustrating the extension of the sustained release up to 35 days [15]. Ruptures of macrophage-rich atherosclerotic plaques in the coronary arteries are the main reason for heart attack. A targeted therapeutic effect on the macrophages will provide a beneficial effect. Receptor-specific targeting using statin-loaded nanometer-sized triblock copolymer vesicles with targeting moieties provides improved efficacy. Vesicle uptake by target cells was observed along with the slow intracellular content release, compared to free drug. No increased cytotoxicity was observed in muscle cells, indicating its promising treatment approach [16].

LIPOSOMES

Liposomes are formed with lipid bilayers possessing the quality of hydrophilicity and hydrophobicity. Based on their size and number of bilayers, liposomes can be of small unilamellar vesicles (SUV) and have a single lipid bilayer; large unilamellar vesicles (LUV) are similar to SUVs, whereas multilamellar vesicles (MLV) have numerous bilayers. With a surface modification of PEG, liposomes are termed as "stealth" having prolonged circulation [3]. The liposomes can be functionalized with functional moieties to reach specific target areas. Dvir *et al.* used angiotensin II type 1 (AT1) liposome to specifically target infarcted heart cardiac cells. His team used nanosized PEGylated liposome carrying a therapeutic payload and conjugated with targeting moiety (amino acid sequence of AT1 receptor), to ensure that nanoparticles are entering into the MI-specific injured mice. The fluorescently labelled nanoparticles were intravenously injected into the right jugular vein of MI mouse model, after 24 h, the mice were sacrificed and hearts were taken out and imaged in an *in vivo* imaging system. The particles were significantly accumulated in MI mouse model and negligibly bound in sham-operated mice (*i.e.,* animals without coronary occlusion) [17]. In another study, anti-P-selectin-conjugated liposomes containing vascular endothelial growth factor (VEGF), was administered to the rat MI model, and the change in cardiac function and vasculature post-MI were quantified. The targeted delivery resulted in a significant increase in fractional shortening and improved systolic function whereas, no significant improvements in cardiac functions were observed in untreated, systemic VEGF-treated, nontargeted liposome-treated, or blank immunoliposome-treated animals [18]. Zhang *et al*. conjugated peptide with an arginine-rich sequence; CRPPR peptide (heart homing peptide), to the liposomes and injected it to MI murine model, which resulted in an increase of fluorescence intensity compared to non-conjugated liposomes and free dye. Due to active targeting mode, the peptide conjugated liposomes were able to target the endothelial lining of the heart and deliver the fluorescent dye across the endothelium [19]. In another study, a stable magnetic nanobead/adenovirus complex was developed for gene-based therapy towards the enhancement of post-infarction myocardial repair under external magnetic control. This complex was administered *via* intravenous injection to ischaemically damaged hearts in a rat acute myocardial infarction model. The placement of epicardial magnet attracted MNBs/ (Ad)–encoded hVEGF gene (Ad_{hVEGF}) complex resulted in better therapeutic gene expression in the ischemic zone of the heart, thereafter, it promoted angiogenesis and improved heart function [20].

DENDRIMERS

Dendrimers are the branched polymers and are one of the promising agents for application in the gene therapy of CVDs, as they possess primary amine end groups that can effectively interact with and biological molecules such as compact DNA plasmids or siRNA by electrostatic interactions and inturn forms nano-composites. Dendrimers that are commonly used in drug delivery are mainly modified in the following three ways: PEGylation; targeting groups, such as folic acid (FA) receptor; and stimuli-sensitive functional groups, sensitive to pH stimuli for lower toxicities, reduced immunogenicities, higher biocompatibilities and better drug-loading capacities. Dendrimers are used for the treatments of MI. Won *et al*. developed a new post-translationally regulated hypoxia-responsible VEGF plasmid, PAM-ABP/VEGF (ABP = arginine-grafted bio-reducible poly (disulfide amine), in which PAM-ABP was a dendrimer-type bio-reducible polymer used as a VEGF carrier. PAM-ABP, could enhance cellular uptake and are less susceptible to reducing agents hence, it resulted in a greater transfection efficiency compared to ABP alone. The dendrimeric VEGF plasmid protected rat cardiomyocytes against apoptosis, preserved their left ventricular (LV) function and prevented LV from remodelling more effectively [21]. Simvastatin (SMV) is a specific inhibitor of HMG -CoA reductase and an effective cholesterol-lowering drug generally used in the clinical setting to treat hypercholesterolemia and reduce coronary events through mechanisms of antioxidant, anti-inflammatory and antiproliferative effects. Kulhari *et al.* constructed three different PAMAM dendrimer (NH_2, OH and PEG)-based and forms SMV nanocomplex for an improvement of the oral absorption of SMV *in vitro* as well as *in vivo*. The formulation showed better pharmacokinetics, and longer SMV residence time. The PAMAM dendrimer formulations illustrated lower plasma cholesterol, reduction of triglycerides and low-density lipoproteins compared to pure SMV [22]. Calcium channel blocking drug nifedipine is used for the treatment of hypotensive and angina patients. Devarakonda *et al.* used generation (G0–G3) of PAMAM dendrimers with both amine and ester termination to intensify its therapeutic concentration for the treatment of CVD by increasing the aqueous solubility of nifedipine at pH of 7, due to the change in the degree of protonation of the dendrimers [23]. Three different conjugates of PAMAM dendrimer and A3 AR agonists, named MRS5216, MRS5246 and MRS5539, showed that these three conjugates protected ischemic rat cardiomyocytes from hypoxia injury and significantly decreased the infarct size in the isolated rat hearts [24]. A study conducted with MRS5246 showed that it was effective in increasing the recovery function of isolated mouse hearts after 20 min of ischemia followed by 45 min of reperfusion, showing significant improvement in the left ventricular developed pressure (LVDP) [25]. PAMAM dendrimers can also serve as a biocompatible polymer, which is able to activate a certain type of adenosine receptors (ARs). Keene *et al.* constructed a new multivalent dendrimeric conjugate of (G5.5 PAMAM dendrimer with an N6-chain-functionalized adenosine agonist) and investigated the cardioprotective effects of activated A3AR on HL-1 cardiomyocytes. They found that this conjugate non-selectively activated the A3AR, inhibited forskolin-stimulated cAMP formation, and protected HL-1 cells from apoptosis induced by H_2O_2 [26]. Dendrimer is also used as a carrier to deliver hypoxia-regulated human VEGF-165 plasmids into skeletal myoblasts (SkMs). These gene-manipulated SkMs were transplanted into infarct myocardium for cardiac repair in a MI model that expresses the VEGF gene. The intramyocardial transplantation of transfected SkMs significantly reduced the apoptotic myocardiocytes, improved the survival of grafted cells, decreased the infarct size, interstitial fibrosis and increased the blood vessel density, which inhibited left ventricle remodeling and improved heart function [27]. Some nanoformulations (polymer, liposomes, dendrimer) that are used for cardiovascular purpose are listed in Table **1**.

Table 1. Some of recent nanoformulations studied for cardiovascular diseases.

Types	Nanoparticle Formulations	Target Region	References
Polymeric			
1	PLGA nanoparticles containing alendronate	Coronary artery	[28]

(Table 1) cont.....

Types	Nanoparticle Formulations	Target Region	References
2	Pitavastatin loaded PLGA nanoformulation	Inhibited plaque destabilization and rupture, reduction of reperfusion injury	[29, 30]
3	Pioglitazone loaded PLGA nanoparticles	Reduction in inflammatory macrophages	[31]
4	PDLLA nanoparticles containing sirolimus	Smooth muscle cells	[32]
5	Hyaluronan nanoparticles	Inhibition in atherosclerotic lesions	[33]
6	Methotraxate-Loaded Hybrid Nanoconstructs	Target vascular Lesions and Inhibit atherosclerosis progression	[34]
7	IL-10 loaded polymeric nanoparticles	Prevents vulnerable plaque in atherosclerosis	[35]
Liposomes			
8	Liposomes containing alendronate	Coronary artery	[36]
9	Lipid-polymeric nanoparticles loaded with paclitaxel	Coronary artery	[37]
10	Colloidal nanoparticles-loaded thrombin	Acute arterial	[38]
11	Ligand-decorated liposome nanoparticles	Activated platelet	[39]
12	HDL covered by liposomes	Aortic cholesterol contents	[40]
13	Liposomal amiodarone	targeted cardiomyocyte	[41]
14	Docetaxel loaded lipid core nanoparticles	Liposomal phenytoin	[42]
15	Liposomal phenytoin	CD43+ inflammatory monocyte for improved left-ventricular function	[43]
16	Amiodarone liposomes	Enhanced cardioprotection effects	[44]
17	Carvedilol Niosome	To enhanced intestinal absorption	[45]
18	Diltiazem Niosome	To enhanced the bioavailability	[46]
Dendrimers			
19	Dendrimer nanoparticles	Localization of ischemic myocardium	[47]
20	Mannose functionalized dendrimeric nanoparticles	Selective delivery to macrophages for atherosclerotic plaques reduction	[48]
21	Nanovector (AT1-PEG-DGL) anchored with AT1 targeting peptide, and with specific microRNA-1 inhibitor (AMO-1)	Reduced cardiomyocyte apoptosis	[49]
Other nanoparticles			
22	Gold-coated immunomicelles	Macrophages in atherosclerosis	[50]
23	Superparamagnetic nanoparticles derived fluorophores	Areas of atheroma	[51]

CONCLUSION

Nanocarriers offer unique advantages in the diagnosis and therapy of CVD. With its characteristics style of action, it can effectively solve the problems of targeting, local drug delivery, controlled release, sustained release, and reduction of toxicity. In addition, nanocarriers implementation for CVDs is in infancy as many more issue still remains unclear. Therefore, rigorous studies need to be carried out to understand the toxic effects towards the cardiovascular system as well as ways to prevent or eliminate possible adverse effects on health. Nevertheless, for effective translational use, deeper understanding and maturation of the developed product is highly required, along with strong regulatory requirements relating to safety, stability, efficacy and Good Manufacturing Practice-compliant production. Further, the potential nanocarriers as the viable clinical product need continuous dialogue and collaboration between experts involved in all stages of development, starting from academia to industry to regulatory bodies.

CONSENT FOR PUBLICATION

Not Applicable.

CONFLICT OF INTEREST

The author confirms that this chapter contents have no conflict of interest.

ACKNOWLEDGEMENT

FD gratefully acknowledges Dept. of Science and Technology, Govt. of India, for the financial grant [SR/WOS-A/LS-448/2017(G)] in the form of women scientist fellowship (WOS-A).

REFERENCES

[1]   Martín Giménez VM, Kassuha DE, Manucha W. Nanomedicine applied to cardiovascular diseases: latest developments. Ther Adv Cardiovasc Dis 2017; 11(4): 133-42.
[http://dx.doi.org/10.1177/1753944717692293] [PMID: 28198204]

[2]   Dormont F, Varna M, Couvreur P. Nanoplumbers: biomaterials to fight cardiovascular diseases. Mater Today 2018; 21(1): 122-43.
[http://dx.doi.org/10.1016/j.mattod.2017.07.008]

[3]   Sahoo SK, Labhasetwar V. Nanotech approaches to drug delivery and imaging. Drug Discov Today 2003; 8(24): 1112-20.
[http://dx.doi.org/10.1016/S1359-6446(03)02903-9] [PMID: 14678737]

[4]   Torchilin VP. PEG-based micelles as carriers of contrast agents for different imaging modalities. Adv Drug Deliv Rev 2002; 54(2): 235-52.
[http://dx.doi.org/10.1016/S0169-409X(02)00019-4] [PMID: 11897148]

[5]   Maeda H, Nakamura H, Fang J. The EPR effect for macromolecular drug delivery to solid tumors:

Improvement of tumor uptake, lowering of systemic toxicity, and distinct tumor imaging *in vivo*. Adv Drug Deliv Rev 2013; 65(1): 71-9.
[http://dx.doi.org/10.1016/j.addr.2012.10.002] [PMID: 23088862]

[6]   Flögel U, Ding Z, Hardung H, *et al*. *in vivo* monitoring of inflammation after cardiac and cerebral ischemia by fluorine magnetic resonance imaging. Circulation 2008; 118(2): 140-8.
[http://dx.doi.org/10.1161/CIRCULATIONAHA.107.737890] [PMID: 18574049]

[7]   Jokerst JV, Lobovkina T, Zare RN, Gambhir SS. Nanoparticle PEGylation for imaging and therapy. Nanomedicine (Lond) 2011; 6(4): 715-28.
[http://dx.doi.org/10.2217/nnm.11.19] [PMID: 21718180]

[8]   Yang H, Zhao F, Li Y, *et al*. VCAM-1-targeted core/shell nanoparticles for selective adhesion and delivery to endothelial cells with lipopolysaccharide-induced inflammation under shear flow and cellular magnetic resonance imaging *In vitro* . Int J Nanomedicine 2013; 8: 1897-906.
[PMID: 23696701]

[9]   Morachis JM, Mahmoud EA, Almutairi A. Physical and chemical strategies for therapeutic delivery by using polymeric nanoparticles. Pharmacol Rev 2012; 64(3): 505-19.
[http://dx.doi.org/10.1124/pr.111.005363] [PMID: 22544864]

[10]   Charoenphol P, Mocherla S, Bouis D, Namdee K, Pinsky DJ, Eniola-Adefeso O. Targeting therapeutics to the vascular wall in atherosclerosis--carrier size matters. Atherosclerosis 2011; 217(2): 364-70.
[http://dx.doi.org/10.1016/j.atherosclerosis.2011.04.016] [PMID: 21601207]

[11]   Buja LM, Vander Heide RS. Pathobiology of ischemic heart disease: past, present and future. Cardiovasc Pathol 2016; 25(3): 214-20.
[http://dx.doi.org/10.1016/j.carpath.2016.01.007] [PMID: 26897485]

[12]   Silva EA, Mooney DJ. Effects of VEGF temporal and spatial presentation on angiogenesis
[http://dx.doi.org/10.1016/j.biomaterials.2009.10.052]

[13]   Davda J, Labhasetwar V. Characterization of nanoparticle uptake by endothelial cells. Int J Pharm 2002; 233(1-2): 51-9.
[http://dx.doi.org/10.1016/S0378-5173(01)00923-1] [PMID: 11897410]

[14]   Panyam J, Labhasetwar V. Biodegradable nanoparticles for drug and gene delivery to cells and tissue. Adv Drug Deliv Rev 2003; 55(3): 329-47.
[http://dx.doi.org/10.1016/S0169-409X(02)00228-4] [PMID: 12628320]

[15]   O'Dwyer J, Murphy R, Dolan EB, *et al*. Development of a nanomedicine-loaded hydrogel for sustained delivery of an angiogenic growth factor to the ischaemic myocardium. Drug Deliv Transl Res 2020; 10(2): 440-54.
[http://dx.doi.org/10.1007/s13346-019-00684-5] [PMID: 31691161]

[16]   Broz P, Ben-Haim N, Grzelakowski M, Marsch S, Meier W, Hunziker P. Inhibition of macrophage phagocytotic activity by a receptor-targeted polymer vesicle-based drug delivery formulation of pravastatin. J Cardiovasc Pharmacol 2008; 51(3): 246-52.
[http://dx.doi.org/10.1097/FJC.0b013e3181624aed] [PMID: 18356688]

[17]   Dvir T, Bauer M, Schroeder A, *et al*. Nanoparticles targeting the infarcted heart. Nano Lett 2011; 11(10): 4411-4.
[http://dx.doi.org/10.1021/nl2025882] [PMID: 21899318]

[18]   Scott RC, Rosano JM, Ivanov Z, *et al*. Targeting VEGF-encapsulated immunoliposomes to MI heart improves vascularity and cardiac function. FASEB J 2009; 23(10): 3361-7.
[http://dx.doi.org/10.1096/fj.08-127373] [PMID: 19535683]

[19]   Zhang H, Li N, Sirish P, *et al*. The cargo of CRPPR-conjugated liposomes crosses the intact murine cardiac endothelium. J Control Release 2012; 163(1): 10-7.
[http://dx.doi.org/10.1016/j.jconrel.2012.06.038] [PMID: 22776291]

[20]   Zhang Y, Li W, Ou L, *et al.* Targeted delivery of human VEGF gene *via* complexes of magnetic nanoparticle-adenoviral vectors enhanced cardiac regeneration. PLoS One 2012; 7(7): e39490.
[http://dx.doi.org/10.1371/journal.pone.0039490] [PMID: 22844395]

[21]   Won YW, McGinn AN, Lee M, Nam K, Bull DA, Kim SW. Post-translational regulation of a hypoxia-responsive VEGF plasmid for the treatment of myocardial ischemia. Biomaterials 2013; 34(26): 6229-38.
[http://dx.doi.org/10.1016/j.biomaterials.2013.04.061] [PMID: 23714244]

[22]   Kulhari H, Kulhari DP, Prajapati SK, Chauhan AS. Pharmacokinetic and pharmacodynamic studies of poly(amidoamine) dendrimer based simvastatin oral formulations for the treatment of hypercholesterolemia. Mol Pharm 2013; 10(7): 2528-33.
[http://dx.doi.org/10.1021/mp300650y] [PMID: 23692066]

[23]   Devarakonda B, Hill RA. The effect of PAMAM dendrimer generation size and surface functional group on the aqueous solubility of nifedipine. Int J Pharm 2004; 284(12): 133-40.

[24]   Chanyshev B, Shainberg A, Isak A, *et al.* Anti-ischemic effects of multivalent dendrimeric A_3 adenosine receptor agonists in cultured cardiomyocytes and in the isolated rat heart. Pharmacol Res 2012; 65(3): 338-46.
[http://dx.doi.org/10.1016/j.phrs.2011.11.013] [PMID: 22154845]

[25]   Wan TC, Tosh DK, Du L, Gizewski ET, Jacobson KA, Auchampach JA. Polyamidoamine (PAMAM) dendrimer conjugate specifically activates the A3 adenosine receptor to improve post-ischemic/reperfusion function in isolated mouse hearts. BMC Pharmacol 2011; 11: 11.
[http://dx.doi.org/10.1186/1471-2210-11-11] [PMID: 22039965]

[26]   Keene AM, Balasubramanian R, Lloyd J, Shainberg A, Jacobson KA. Multivalent dendrimeric and monomeric adenosine agonists attenuate cell death in HL-1 mouse cardiomyocytes expressing the A(3) receptor. Biochem Pharmacol 2010; 80(2): 188-96.
[http://dx.doi.org/10.1016/j.bcp.2010.03.020] [PMID: 20346920]

[27]   Zhu K, Guo C, Xia Y, *et al.* Transplantation of novel vascular endothelial growth factor gene delivery system manipulated skeletal myoblasts promote myocardial repair. Int J Cardiol 2013; 168(3): 2622-31.
[http://dx.doi.org/10.1016/j.ijcard.2013.03.041] [PMID: 23578891]

[28]   Cohen-Sela E, Chorny M, Koroukhov N, Danenberg HD, Golomb G. A new double emulsion solvent diffusion technique for encapsulating hydrophilic molecules in PLGA nanoparticles. J Control Release 2009; 133(2): 90-5.
[http://dx.doi.org/10.1016/j.jconrel.2008.09.073] [PMID: 18848962]

[29]   Ichimura K, Matoba T, Nakano K, *et al.* A Translational Study of a New Therapeutic Approach for Acute Myocardial Infarction: Nanoparticle-Mediated Delivery of Pitavastatin into Reperfused Myocardium Reduces Ischemia-Reperfusion Injury in a Preclinical Porcine Model. PLoS One 2016; 11(9): e0162425.
[http://dx.doi.org/10.1371/journal.pone.0162425] [PMID: 27603665]

[30]   Katsuki S, Matoba T, Nakashiro S, *et al.* Nanoparticle-mediated delivery of pitavastatin inhibits atherosclerotic plaque destabilization/rupture in mice by regulating the recruitment of inflammatory monocytes. Circulation 2014; 129(8): 896-906.
[http://dx.doi.org/10.1161/CIRCULATIONAHA.113.002870] [PMID: 24305567]

[31]   Nakashiro S, Matoba T, Umezu R, *et al.* Pioglitazone-incorporated nanoparticles prevent plaque destabilization and rupture by regulating monocyte/macrophage differentiation in apoe −/− mice. Arterioscler Thromb Vasc Biol 2016; 36(3): 491-500.
[http://dx.doi.org/10.1161/ATVBAHA.115.307057] [PMID: 26821947]

[32]   Zhao J, Mo Z, Guo F, Shi D, Han QQ, Liu Q. Drug loaded nanoparticle coating on totally bioresorbable PLLA stents to prevent in-stent restenosis. J Biomed Mater Res B Appl Biomater 2018; 106(1): 88-95.

[http://dx.doi.org/10.1002/jbm.b.33794] [PMID: 27875036]

[33]   Beldman TJ, Senders ML, Alaarg A, *et al.* Hyaluronan nanoparticles selectively target plaque-associated macrophages and improve plaque stability in atherosclerosis. ACS Nano 2017; 11(6): 5785-99.
[http://dx.doi.org/10.1021/acsnano.7b01385] [PMID: 28463501]

[34]   Stigliano C, Ramirez MR, Singh JV, *et al.* Methotraxate-loaded hybrid nanoconstructs target vascular lesions and inhibit atherosclerosis progression in apoe-/- mice. Adv Healthc Mater 2017; 6(13): 1601286.
[http://dx.doi.org/10.1002/adhm.201601286] [PMID: 28402587]

[35]   Kamaly N, Fredman G, Fojas JJR, *et al.* Targeted interleukin-10 nanotherapeutics developed with a microfluidic chip enhance resolution of inflammation in advanced atherosclerosis. ACS Nano 2016; 10(5): 5280-92.
[http://dx.doi.org/10.1021/acsnano.6b01114] [PMID: 27100066]

[36]   Gutman D, Golomb G. Liposomal alendronate for the treatment of restenosis. J Control Release 2012; 161(2): 619-27.
[http://dx.doi.org/10.1016/j.jconrel.2011.11.037] [PMID: 22178594]

[37]   Chan JM, Rhee JW, Drum CL, *et al.* in vivo prevention of arterial restenosis with paclitaxel-encapsulated targeted lipid-polymeric nanoparticles. Proc Natl Acad Sci USA 2011; 108(48): 19347-52.
[http://dx.doi.org/10.1073/pnas.1115945108] [PMID: 22087004]

[38]   Myerson J, He L, Lanza G, Tollefsen D, Wickline S. Thrombin-inhibiting perfluorocarbon nanoparticles provide a novel strategy for the treatment and magnetic resonance imaging of acute thrombosis. J Thromb Haemost 2011; 9(7): 1292-300.
[http://dx.doi.org/10.1111/j.1538-7836.2011.04339.x] [PMID: 21605330]

[39]   Srinivasan R, Marchant RE, Gupta AS. *In vitro* and *in vivo* platelet targeting by cyclic RGD-modified liposomes. J Biomed Mater Res A 2010; 93(3): 1004-15.
[PMID: 19743511]

[40]   Cho BHS, Park J-R, Nakamura MT, Odintsov BM, Wallig MA, Chung B-H. Synthetic dimyristoylphosphatidylcholine liposomes assimilating into high-density lipoprotein promote regression of atherosclerotic lesions in cholesterol-fed rabbits. Exp Biol Med (Maywood) 2010; 235(10): 1194-203.
[http://dx.doi.org/10.1258/ebm.2010.009320] [PMID: 20876082]

[41]   Zhuge Y, Zheng Z-F, Xie M-Q, Li L, Wang F, Gao F. Preparation of liposomal amiodarone and investigation of its cardiomyocyte-targeting ability in cardiac radiofrequency ablation rat model. Int J Nanomedicine 2016; 11: 2359-67.
[http://dx.doi.org/10.2147/IJN.S98815] [PMID: 27313453]

[42]   Meneghini BC, Tavares ER, Guido MC, *et al.* Lipid core nanoparticles as vehicle for docetaxel reduces atherosclerotic lesion, inflammation, cell death and proliferation in an atherosclerosis rabbit model. Vascul Pharmacol 2019; 115: 46-54.
[http://dx.doi.org/10.1016/j.vph.2019.02.003] [PMID: 30797043]

[43]   Zhou X, Luo Y-C, Ji W-J, *et al.* Modulation of mononuclear phagocyte inflammatory response by liposome-encapsulated voltage gated sodium channel inhibitor ameliorates myocardial ischemia/reperfusion injury in rats. PLoS One 2013; 8(9): e74390.
[http://dx.doi.org/10.1371/journal.pone.0074390] [PMID: 24069305]

[44]   Takahama H, Shigematsu H, Asai T, *et al.* Liposomal amiodarone augments anti-arrhythmic effects and reduces hemodynamic adverse effects in an ischemia/reperfusion rat model. Cardiovasc Drugs Ther 2013; 27(2): 125-32.
[http://dx.doi.org/10.1007/s10557-012-6437-6] [PMID: 23344929]

[45]   Arzani G, Haeri A, Daeihamed M, Bakhtiari-Kaboutaraki H, Dadashzadeh S. Niosomal carriers

enhance oral bioavailability of carvedilol: effects of bile salt-enriched vesicles and carrier surface charge. Int J Nanomedicine 2015; 10: 4797-813.
[PMID: 26251598]

[46]   Ammar HO, Haider M, Ibrahim M, El Hoffy NM. *In vitro* and *in vivo* investigation for optimization of niosomal ability for sustainment and bioavailability enhancement of diltiazem after nasal administration. Drug Deliv 2017; 24(1): 414-21.
[http://dx.doi.org/10.1080/10717544.2016.1259371] [PMID: 28165822]

[47]   Magruder JT, Crawford TC, Lin YA, *et al.* Selective Localization of a Novel Dendrimer Nanoparticle in Myocardial Ischemia-Reperfusion Injury. Ann Thorac Surg 2017; 104(3): 891-8.
[http://dx.doi.org/10.1016/j.athoracsur.2016.12.051] [PMID: 28366468]

[48]   He H, Yuan Q, Bie J, *et al.* Development of mannose functionalized dendrimeric nanoparticles for targeted delivery to macrophages: use of this platform to modulate atherosclerosis. Transl Res 2018; 193: 13-30.
[http://dx.doi.org/10.1016/j.trsl.2017.10.008] [PMID: 29172034]

[49]   Xue X, Shi X, Dong H, *et al.* Delivery of microRNA-1 inhibitor by dendrimer-based nanovector: An early targeting therapy for myocardial infarction in mice. Nanomedicine (Lond) 2018; 14(2): 619-31.
[http://dx.doi.org/10.1016/j.nano.2017.12.004] [PMID: 29269324]

[50]   Lipinski MJ, Amirbekian V, Frias JC, *et al.* MRI to detect atherosclerosis with gadolinium-containing immunomicelles targeting the macrophage scavenger receptor. Magn Reson Med 2006; 56(3): 601-10.
[http://dx.doi.org/10.1002/mrm.20995] [PMID: 16902977]

[51]   Stein-Merlob AF, Hara T, McCarthy JR, *et al.* Atheroma Susceptible to Thrombosis Exhibit Impaired Endothelial Permeability *in vivo* as Assessed by Nanoparticle-Based Fluorescence Molecular Imaging. Circ Cardiovasc Imaging 2017; 10(5): e005813.
[http://dx.doi.org/10.1161/CIRCIMAGING.116.005813] [PMID: 28487316]

CHAPTER 6

Nanocarriers for Theranostics Delivery of Cardiovascular Diseases

Pooja Jain[1], Nazia Hassan[1], Manvi Singh[1] and Zeenat Iqbal[1,*]

[1] Nanomedicine Laboratory, School of Pharmaceutical Education and Research, Jamia Hamdard, New Delhi-110062, India

Abstract: Cardiovascular diseases (CVDs), predominant global disabilities, are solely responsible for causing a significant number of deaths annually. The arising issues of conventional therapeutics, such as high insufficiency in reducing disease progression, unpleasant side effects, *etc.,* have made CVDs a significant clinical challenge. Henceforth, the exploration of newer technologies and strategies for CVD management has become a need of present times. Recently, CVDs have become a major area of focus for medical, scientific and technological development. One such area of particular interest is an advancement of nanoparticle drug delivery systems for targeting CVDs, which offers a bouquet of positive attributes such as a high - targeted approach for specific disease sites, drug bioavailability and functional payloads. The present article mainly emphasis on the growing concept of 'theranostic nanoparticles or nanotheranostics' in the field of CVDs. The term 'Theranostic' combinedly refers to the union of diagnostics and therapeutics, with the purpose of enhancing the safety and efficacy of the treatment. Although it is still in its infancy stage for cardiovascular complications, the idea of theranostics has already been applied in the field of oncology and is giving fruitful results as well. The present chapter gives its description in the field of diagnosis as well as therapeutics, which may improve the status of nanomedical research in CVDs.

Keywords: Drug delivery, Nanomedicine, Nanoparticles, Nanotheranostics, Theranostics.

INTRODUCTION

Theranostics is a novel approach to clinical medicine that combines therapeutics and diagnostics with the purpose of enhancing the safety and efficacy of the treatment, such as nanoparticle drug delivery systems (NDDS) [1]. In simple terms, theranostics can be defined as an advanced diagnostic process that is

* **Corresponding author Zeenat Iqbal:**Nanomedicine Laboratory, School of Pharmaceutical Education and Research, Jamia Hamdard, New Delhi-110062, India; Tel: +91-11-26058689-5662, Fax: 011-26059663,
E-mail: zeenatiqbal@jamiahamdard.ac.in

equipped with a therapeutic moiety (drug)/device for improving site-specific targeted approach, drug bioavailability/safety/efficacy, functional payloads and to reduce the related steps and incurred costs of the treatment. Presently, theranostics have garnered wide acceptability and expectations for medical, scientific and technological development because of its multipronged approach [2]. In nanotheranostics, nanoparticles can themselves act as diagnostic probes (imaging/contrast agent) and get conjugated with therapeutic or diagnostic molecules/moiety or vice versa; thus, they can be cited as one of the best examples of theranostics (Fig. **1**).

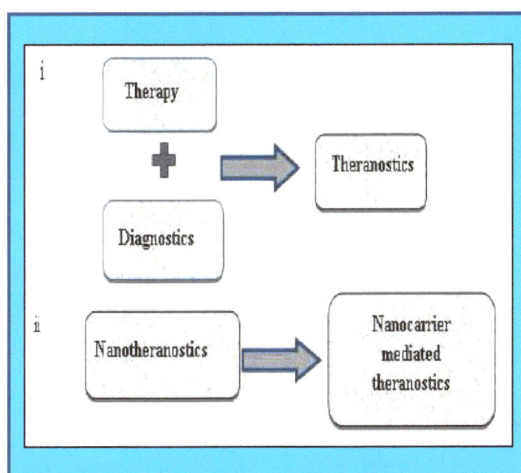

Fig. (1). (i) The model describes the combination of therapy and diagnostic leading to the formation of thernostics **(ii)** the nanotheranostics can be used with *via* nanocarriers.

The advancement of nanobased therapeutics has garnered worldwide attention in major disciplines, such as engineering, chemistry, biology, pharmaceutical science and medicine. Moreover, the synergistic combination of a nanoparticulate approach with theranostics has yielded a novel premise for research and development in the aforementioned field, which is known as 'Nanotheranostics'. Presently, it is cited as a multidisciplinary as well as multipronged approach owing to its great potentials in the field of human healthcare and well-being. It also has played a prominent role in disease treatment and its characterization *via* the development of various biomarkers and personalized medicines. The novel approach of theranostics nanoparticles allows for the simultaneous determination of drug localization, release and efficacy in a variety of conditions such as atherosclerosis [2]. Atherosclerosis is a prevalent cardiovascular complication that can only be detected after the onset of clinical symptoms; hence there is an emerging need to diagnose as well as to treat it as early as possible. The various targets for imaging the plaques are endothelia, fibrin, macrophages as well as various markers of angiogenesis. In atherosclerosis, theranostics nanoparticles imaging capabilities validate the drug to reach the targeted site of action and screen its effect on a molecular level. It also designs dosage regimens and identifies the population that responds to a particular therapy [2]. Although the concept of theranostics has not been applied too much in cardiovascular complications in the near future, it may yield excellent results in the diagnosis as well as therapeutics, which may improve the status of nanomedical research. The 3 verticals of the theranostics nano-approach (Fig. **2**) are introduced below.

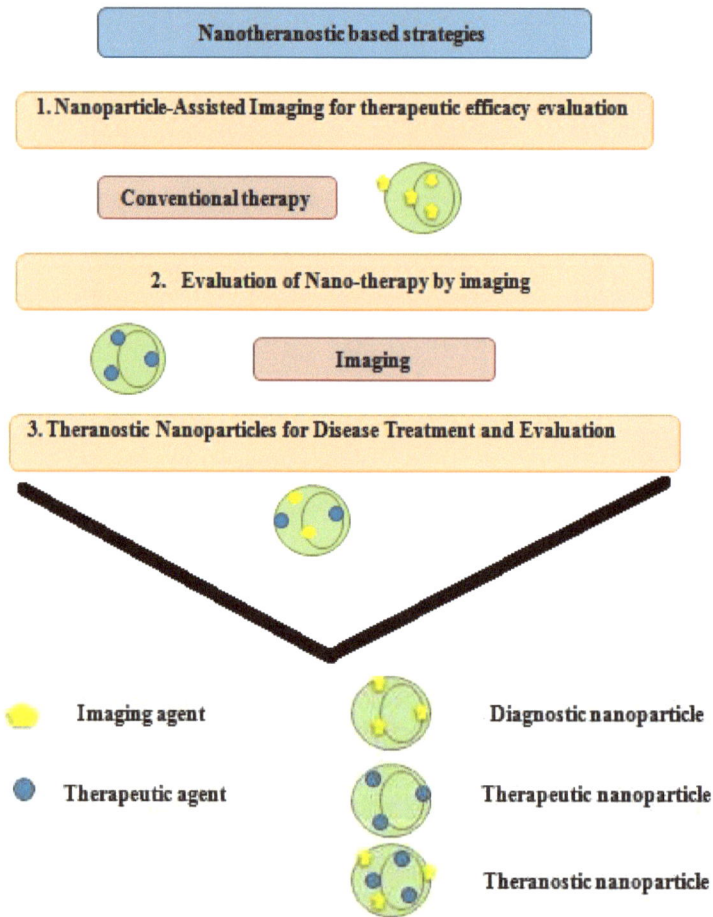

Fig. (2). Outlines of nanotheranostic based approach.

THERANOSTICS IN NANOMEDICINAL RESEARCH

Nanoparticles (NPs) are a widely known nanosized particulate system having wide applications for various diseases. The combination of NP with theranostics opens up a wide array of research owing to its high no. of positive attributes. One of the most intriguing & growing properties of theranostics nanoparticles is their ability to work as an imaging agent by simultaneously incorporating and delivering functional/therapeutic payloads of the treatment. NP with the aforementioned feature is classified as theranostics nanoparticles/ nanotheranostics because of its combined therapeutic and diagnostic functions in a single particulate system. Such property of NP enables disease-related imaging interventions, targeted delivery of therapeutic agent & direct screening of its [absorption, distribution, metabolism & excretion (ADME)] profile and biologic effects [3]. Quite recently, various studies have highlighted the exploitation of theranostics nanoparticles against multiple cardiovascular complications as (i) Stabilization of atheroma's by delivering antiangiogenic and anti-inflammatory drugs, (ii) Delivery of angiogenic factors & genes to treat peripheral artery disease and to promote postinfarct cardiac repair respectively, (iii) Tracking the activity of therapeutic cells delivered to the infarcted myocardium. In CVD, nanoimaging is comparatively a newly introduced area of research as compared to nanomedicinal approach. Such imaging property enables NPs to synergistically improve both diagnostic and therapeutic specificity and efficacy. One such known example of this approach is simultaneous detection and volume reduction of thrombus in cases of thrombolysis/fibrinolysis. A study was conceptualised for the use of iron oxide nanoparticles tagged with recombinant tissue plasminogen activator to efficiently dissolve the clot. Another study was conducted to explore the real-time monitoring of thrombolytic effect using fluorophores coated NPs. Therefore, it can be inferred that diagnosis and reduction of plaque and its volume can be carried out simultaneously *via* nanotheranostics [4].

NANOCARRIERS FOR THERANOSTICS DELIVERY OF CVD

Various CVDs that has been targeted *via* the nanocarriers approach are given below:

ATHEROSCLEROSIS

In both animals and humans, it is well known that the macrophages of atherosclerotic plaques selectively uptakes the ultra-small particles of iron-oxide (USPIO). Moris *et al.* explored the use of USPIO with an improved MRI towards assessing the efficacy of a p38 kinase inhibitor in an apolipoprotein E-deficient mouse model. An *ex-vivo* study showed that all the USPIOs were infiltrated inside the macrophages. Whereas, the MRI study of the aortic arch and root confirmed the reduced deposition of USPIO. Their study revealed the USPIO-enhanced MRI as the non-invasive potential tool for evaluation of therapeutic effects [5]. For the very first time, this method has been used by Tang *et al.* to evaluate the efficacy of high as well as low doses of atorvastatin in patients with carotid plaque inflammation. A marked reduction of USPIO uptake in carotid plaque was observed with high dose treatment after 12 weeks whereas, no such effects were observed with the low dose treatment [6]. Therefore, the USPIO-improved MRI technique can be considered a useful imaging tool for screening atherosclerotic lesions and simultaneous evaluation of therapeutic efficacies of "anti-inflammatory" interventions.

PERIPHERAL ARTERY DISEASE

Peripheral artery disease (PAD) comprises the narrowing of the lumen of peripheral arteries, which then leads to low blood and oxygen supply to the tissue, resulting in critical limb ischemia. By improving blood flow and oxygenation, arteriogenesis, a natural process, has a potential role in minimizing PAD symptoms. And L-arginine can increase arteriogenesis. Winter *et al.* study the neovascular response to angiogenic therapy with alpha (nu)beta (3)-integri--targeted perfluorocarbon nanoparticles in a rabbit model. With *in-vivo* nanoparticle improved MRI, prominent signal enhancement was seen in ischemic hind limbs, which was further confirmed by *ex-vivo* X-ray angiography [7]. There is a possibility that this approach may lead to a prior and more precise detection of treatment generated collateral vessel growth in PAD patients. Therapeutic angiogenesis is a novel and attractive intervention for the treatment of tissue ischemia, involving the delivery of tissue growth factors such as vascular endothelial growth factor (VEGF). However, poor circulatory half-life and no specific targeting limit their clinical use. Studies were performed by the researchers to explore the potential of nanoparticles to increase the therapeutic efficacy of bioactive molecules by improving their circulatory half-life and specificity. In a study performed by Kim *et al.*, VEGF bonded gold nanoparticles were selectively targeted to the ischemic tissue and enhanced therapeutic angiogenesis was achieved. Further, in a murine hind limb model, Laser Doppler imaging of ischemic tissue showed 1.7 times increased perfusion of VEGF-conjugated gold nanoparticles as compared to free VEGF [8].

MINIMIZING REPERFUSION INJURY IN ACUTE MYOCARDIAL INFARCTION

Clinical trials have represented adenosine as a cardio-protectant as an advancement to reperfusion therapy for acute myocardial infarction. But adenosine is associated with a very poor half-life (1-2 second) and severe adverse effects like hypotension and bradycardia. To cater to this issue, Takahama *et al.*, formulated and intravenously injected PEGylated liposomal adenosine to an ischemic/ reperfusion myocardial rat model before the onset of reperfusion. Better myocardial accumulation of liposomes was observed in infarcted areas as observed through transmission electron microscopy and *ex vivo* bioluminescence. Further, better response in terms of improved half-life, minimal adverse effects and reduced myocardial infarction size was observed with the liposomal adenosine as compared to the free adenosine [9].

THROMBOSIS TREATMENTS

Localized thrombosis in the lumen of the coronary artery is the origin of heart attack and is conventionally treated with a combination of a variety of anti-coagulants and anti-platelet agents given orally and intravenously. But despite high dose regimens, thrombus formation exceeds unpredictably. Myerson *et al*. demonstrated that a perfluoro-carbon core-nanoparticle covalently attached with an irreversible thrombin inhibitor *i.e* D-phenylalanyl-l-prolyl -l-arginyl-chloro methyl ketone (PPACK) offered a safer and more successful approach for localized antithrombotic effect and simultaneously serves as an imaging tool to detect an acute thrombosis in the artery or vein as their ability to be imaged through magnetic resonance imaging (MRI) and spectroscopy of its fluorine (19F) core [10]. In a similar study, Peters *et al*. developed modular multi-functional micelles, containing a fluorophore, an anti-coagulation component and a peptide that is specifically attached to clotted plasma proteins. *Ex-vivo* fluorescence imaging showed specific *in-vivo* targeting of nanomicelles to atherosclerotic plaques. In ApoEKO mice, better results were obtained when hirulog anti-thrombosis peptide is loaded on micelles as compared to free hirulog at the same molar concentration [11].

VASCULAR INJURY AND STENOSIS INHIBITION

Due to atherosclerotic progression, luminal narrowing of the blood vessels takes place and this is called as stenosis. In order to revascularize the stenotic vessels, balloon dilation and stent placement are the two preferred approaches. However, other complications like myocardial infarction and poor peripheral circulation may results due to restenosis in dilated and stented vessels. Although drug-eluting stents can minimize in-stent restenosis but can also disturb the endothelial healing, which may lead to late-stent thrombosis. Chorny *et al*. formulated paclitaxel loaded magnetic nanoparticles and explored the magnetic property of stents. After application of magnetic field upon administration, drug-loaded magnetic nanoparticles specifically gathered in the stented areas and a high concentration of paclitaxel was achieved. Fluorescence imaging and histology confirm that local accumulation of MNPs had delayed the cell proliferation and in-stent restenosis [12]. They concluded that the improved therapeutic effects were obtained after application of magnetic field and simultaneously, local drug concentration can be adjusted by monitoring the external magnetic field.

INHIBITING RESTENOSIS

As stated earlier, revascularization treatment is frequently followed by restenosis. It is believed that the proliferation of smooth muscle cell (SMC) in the walls of artery/vein, promote restenosis and attempts has been made by the researchers to develop strategies to inhibit restenosis. Lanza *et al.*, develop perfluorocarbon nanoparticles of anti-proliferation drugs doxorubicin and paclitaxel and deliver to SMC in the arterial wall of restenotic vessels. SMCs were targeted by the nanoparticles and *in-vitro* inhibition of tissue proliferation was observed. 19F MRI spectroscopy helped to differentiate the nanoparticles from other tissues, whereas T1-weighted MRI detected the selective uptake of particles [13]. Their study proposed a novel theranostic nanoparticle-based system for cardiovascular disease.

STABILIZING HIGH-RISK ATHEROSCLEROTIC PLAQUES

It is well established that the inhibition of angiogenesis slows down the progress of atherosclerosis. To validate the fact, Winter *et al.*, targeted the $\alpha v\beta 3$-integrin with the paramagnetic nanoparticles of anti-angiogenesis drug fumagillin. Response to treatment in terms of changes in signal enhancement in atherosclerotic plaque was measured by MRI. After treatment, the signal enhancement was decreased, illustrating reduced angiogenesis. *Ex-vivo* staining of microvessels was used to evaluate the *in-vivo* activity. Their study presented the dual-purpose theranostic nanoparticles as a potential candidate for atherosclerosis [14]. In another study, McCarthy *et al.* targeted macrophages with the theranostic nanoparticles. Dextran-coated iron-oxide nanoparticles were developed and loaded with near-infrared fluorophores and phototoxic agents. Macrophages were specifically targeted and activated by the nanoparticles and light respectively to induce apoptosis. Intravital fluorescence microscopy was performed in an ApoE KO mouse model, and it was observed that nanoparticles were selectively localized in the atherosclerotic plaques. *Ex-vivo* histology showed that the nanoparticles induced massive destruction of macrophages and minimal skin toxicity than free phototoxic agents [15].

CONCLUSION

The wide popularity and approachability of nanotheranostics are due to its dual approach in terms of diagnosis and therapy in a variety of diseases, especially cancer. Such an approach enables enhanced disease imaging, personalized/targeted treatment, improved therapeutics safety, efficacy, bioavailability and functional payloads. In CVDs, the application of nanotheranostics has been preclinically applied and has yielded several interesting and encouraging findings as well. However, despite such tremendous progress, the concept of nanotheranostics still requires broader attention in order to open a brand-new avenue for tailored as well as personalized patient care against various life-threatening human diseases.

CONSENT FOR PUBLICATION

Not Applicable.

CONFLICT OF INTEREST

The author confirms that this chapter contents have no conflict of interest.

ACKNOWLEDGEMENT

Pooja Jain is thankful to Jamia Hamdard for providing Jamia Hamdard-Silver Jubilee research fellowship-2017, AS/Fellow/JH-5/2018.

REFERENCES

[1]   Bejarano J, Navarro-Marquez M, Morales-Zavala F, *et al.* Nanoparticles for diagnosis and therapy of atherosclerosis and myocardial infarction: evolution toward prospective theranostic approaches. Theranostics 2018; 8(17): 4710-32.
[http://dx.doi.org/10.7150/thno.26284] [PMID: 30279733]

[2]   Cattaneo M, Froio A, Gallino A. Cardiovascular Imaging and Theranostics in Cardiovascular Pharmacotherapy. Eur Cardiol 2019; 14(1): 62-4.
[http://dx.doi.org/10.15420/ecr.2019.6.1] [PMID: 31131039]

[3]   Juenet M, Varna M, Chauvierre C, Letourneur D. Nanotheranostics in cardiovascular diseases. 2016.
[http://dx.doi.org/10.1142/9789814713535_0009]

[4]   Flores AM, Ye J, Jarr K-U, Hosseini-Nassab N, Smith BR, Leeper NJ. Nanoparticle therapy for vascular diseases. Arterioscler Thromb Vasc Biol 2019; 39(4): 635-46.
[http://dx.doi.org/10.1161/ATVBAHA.118.311569] [PMID: 30786744]

[5]   Morris JB, Olzinski AR, Bernard RE, *et al.* p38 MAPK inhibition reduces aortic ultrasmall superparamagnetic iron oxide uptake in a mouse model of atherosclerosis: MRI assessment. Arterioscler Thromb Vasc Biol 2008; 28(2): 265-71.
[http://dx.doi.org/10.1161/ATVBAHA.107.151175] [PMID: 18162612]

[6]   Tang TY, Howarth SPS, Miller SR, *et al.* The ATHEROMA (Atorvastatin Therapy: Effects on Reduction of Macrophage Activity) Study. Evaluation using ultrasmall superparamagnetic iron oxide-enhanced magnetic resonance imaging in carotid disease. J Am Coll Cardiol 2009; 53(22): 2039-50.
[http://dx.doi.org/10.1016/j.jacc.2009.03.018] [PMID: 19477353]

[7]   Winter PM, Caruthers SD, Allen JS, *et al.* Molecular imaging of angiogenic therapy in peripheral vascular disease with alphanubeta3-integrin-targeted nanoparticles. Magn Reson Med 2010; 64(2): 369-76.
[http://dx.doi.org/10.1002/mrm.22447] [PMID: 20665780]

[8]   Kim J, Cao L, Shvartsman D, Silva EA, Mooney DJ. Targeted delivery of nanoparticles to ischemic muscle for imaging and therapeutic angiogenesis. Nano Lett 2011; 11(2): 694-700.
[http://dx.doi.org/10.1021/nl103812a] [PMID: 21192718]

[9]   Takahama H, Minamino T, Asanuma H, *et al.* Prolonged targeting of ischemic/reperfused myocardium

by liposomal adenosine augments cardioprotection in rats. J Am Coll Cardiol 2009; 53(8): 709-17.
[http://dx.doi.org/10.1016/j.jacc.2008.11.014] [PMID: 19232905]

[10] Myerson J, He L, Lanza G, Tollefsen D, Wickline S. Thrombin-inhibiting perfluorocarbon nanoparticles provide a novel strategy for the treatment and magnetic resonance imaging of acute thrombosis. J Thromb Haemost 2011; 9(7): 1292-300.
[http://dx.doi.org/10.1111/j.1538-7836.2011.04339.x] [PMID: 21605330]

[11] Peters D, Kastantin M, Kotamraju VR, *et al.* Targeting atherosclerosis by using modular, multifunctional micelles. Proc Natl Acad Sci USA 2009; 106(24): 9815-9.
[http://dx.doi.org/10.1073/pnas.0903369106] [PMID: 19487682]

[12] Chorny M, Fishbein I, Yellen BB, *et al.* Targeting stents with local delivery of paclitaxel-loaded magnetic nanoparticles using uniform fields. Proc Natl Acad Sci USA 2010; 107(18): 8346-51.
[http://dx.doi.org/10.1073/pnas.0909506107] [PMID: 20404175]

[13] Lanza GM, Winter PM, Caruthers SD, *et al.* Theragnostics for tumor and plaque angiogenesis with perfluorocarbon nanoemulsions. Angiogenesis 2010; 13(2): 189-202.
[http://dx.doi.org/10.1007/s10456-010-9166-0] [PMID: 20411320]

[14] Winter PM, Neubauer AM, Caruthers SD, *et al.* Endothelial $\alpha(v)\beta3$ integrin-targeted fumagillin nanoparticles inhibit angiogenesis in atherosclerosis. Arterioscler Thromb Vasc Biol 2006; 26(9): 2103-9.
[http://dx.doi.org/10.1161/01.ATV.0000235724.11299.76] [PMID: 16825592]

[15] McCarthy JR, Korngold E, Weissleder R, Jaffer FA. A light-activated theranostic nanoagent for targeted macrophage ablation in inflammatory atherosclerosis. Small 2010; 6(18): 2041-9.
[http://dx.doi.org/10.1002/smll.201000596] [PMID: 20721949]

CHAPTER 7

Nanocarriers for Biologicals Delivery to Cardiovascular System

Fahima Dilnawaz[1],*

[1] *Laboratory of Nanomedicine, Institute of Life Sciences, Nalco Square, Chandrasekharpur, Bhubaneswar-751023, Odisha, India*

Abstract: As cardiovascular diseases remain the leading cause of mortality worldwide, a large number of clinical trials are under development, investigating the safety and efficacy of RNA therapeutics in clinical conditions. Nanomedicine based drug delivery systems are currently the new avenue for the treatment of CVDs, providing great advantages to the treatment regime of CVDs. Currently, antisense therapy DNA- and RNA-based and microRNAs are widely applied therapeutic strategies to regulate gene expression and its effect on CVDs. In this review, different biological-based targeting therapies for cardiovascular diseases and their outcomes are discussed.

Keywords: DNA, miRNA, Nanomedicine, Nanoparticles, RNA interference, siRNA.

INTRODUCTION

Cardiovascular diseases are the leading cause of death and disability, surpassing infectious diseases due to lifestyle changes in developing as well as developed countries. Prescribed medicines do provide enormous benefits to the patients, but the adverse effect on the kidney and liver can never be negated. In this regard, advanced studies in RNA biology have been achieved with the help of microRNAs and short interfering RNAs, which regulate various cellular processes across the eukaryotes. RNA interference (RNAi) offers the possibility to silence every defectively expressed gene in a given disease. The structural similarities of siRNA and miRNA have been well explored for cardiovascular disease applications. In the mammalian system, the miRNAs are encoded in the genome, processed in the nucleus by the cell of origin, whereas siRNAs are exogenously delivered.

---

* **Corresponding author Fahima Dilnawaz:** Laboratory of Nanomedicine, Institute of Life Sciences, Nalco Square, Chandrasekharpur, Bhubaneswar 751023, India; Tel: +91-674 – 2304341, 2304283, Fax: 91-674-2300728; E-mail: fahimadilnawaz@gmail.com

While siRNAs lead to degradation of target mRNA, miRNAs lead to either degradation or translational inhibition of target mRNA (Fig. **1**).

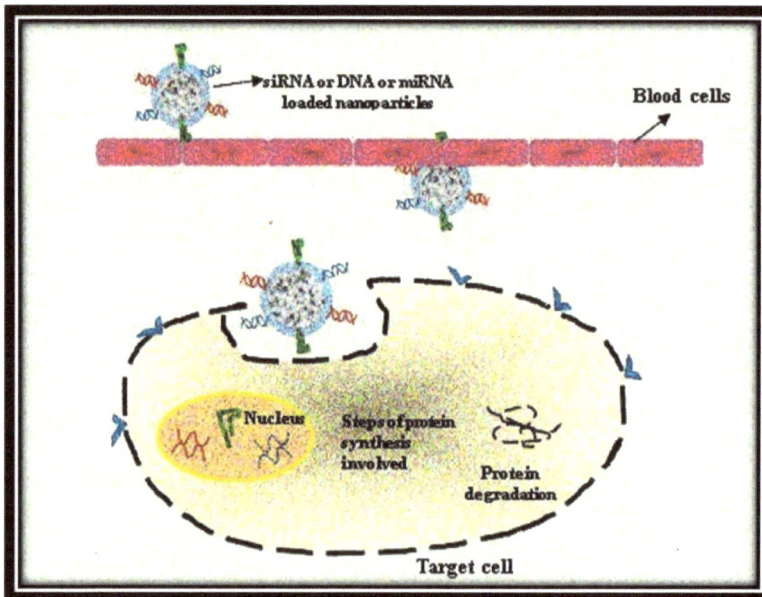

Fig. (1). General process of entry of siRNA, DNA or miRNA through the blood vessels to the target cells and degradation of its target protein.

Systemic delivery of siRNA nanovehicles has been explored for cardiovascular disease applications. Nanomaterials-based delivery of siRNA (or miRNA) hold great promise for gene therapy in cardiac diseases. For cardiac application, siRNA (or miRNA) therapy-based cardiac targeting still remains an issue, and several strategies are used for the improvement of cardiac uptake. siRNA (or miRNA) therapy strategies are used for the improvement of cardiovascular disease with encouraging results. A growing understanding of cardiac science can open up new facets for the successful functioning of siRNA and miRNA for better therapeutic outcomes. With the help of suitably designed siRNA, the RNAi machinery can be utilized for silencing any gene in the body and providing a better therapeutic effect than other typical small drug molecules [1]. Various studies have documented the efficacy of the synthetic siRNA's knocking down targets *in vivo* . Therefore, methods are applied to target only the cardiovascular system, which has shown minimal side effects. But for achieving the desired clinical outcomes, a safe and effective delivery system for siRNA is of paramount importance. Over the last decades, progress in nanotechnology has been implemented to develop nanomedicine for CVD therapies. A variety of nanoparticles-based formulations have been developed containing drugs, proteins, and biologics have been tested pre-clinically to provide some encouraging results for cardiovascular-specific applications, such as hypercholesterolaemia [2], hepatitis [3], liver cirrhosis [4], bone cancer [5] and ovarian cancer [6].

SIRNA BASED APPLICATIONS

Small interference RNA (siRNA) technology effectively attenuates specific proteins *in vivo* by the degradation of mRNA [7]. However, siRNA being a large molecule with a negative charge faces problems while crossing the cell membrane [8]. To combat these challenges, nanoparticles mediated delivery vehicle is chosen. Various delivery systems have been developed for targeting the siRNA in cardiovascular diseases. Li *et al.* developed an amino-acid based nanoparticle HB-OLD 7 for local delivery of siRNA targeting NOX2 to the arterial wall. In an atherosclerotic rat model after angioplasty, the siRNA nanoparticles were successfully transferred into regional carotid artery walls. The Cybb gene expression was reduced to > 87% compared to angioplastic controls [9]. In another study, Frank-Kamenetsky, Maria *et al.* developed cross-species, siRNA proprotein convertase subtilins/kexin type 9 (PCSK9) and targeted it to non-human primate-like murine rat. PCSK9 regulates low-density lipoprotein receptor (LDLR). For the study, they formulated siRNA lipidoid nanoparticles and studied their targeting efficacy in mice and rat models. The liver-specific siRNA silencing decreases the PCSK9 mRNA levels by ~ 50-70% that is associated with a reduction in plasma cholesterol concentration of ~ 60%. They suggested that the targeting of PCSK9 can be a treatment strategy for hypercholesterolemia treatment [2]. Gene silencing stent is a promising approach for regeneration of vascular endothelial cell wall and inhibition of restenosis. Gene silencing stents consist of specific siRNAs which are released to the vascular endothelial cell wall. For combating coronary diseases, Hossfeld *et al.* developed a layer-by-layer technology of multilayers of chitosan and hyaluronic acid (HA) nanoparticles. The coated stents were evaluated in an ex-vivo model with porcine carotid arteries, which provoked the uptake of siRNA /chitosan nanoparticles into the artery walls and long-term siRNA release, illustrating it as a powerful technique to prevent restenosis [10]. Silencing C-C chemokine receptor type 2 (CCR2) provides cellular specificity for this emerging therapeutic target. Therefore, the use of nanoparticles can be an effective strategy for siRNA to prevent the inflammatory cycle of atherosclerosis. Monocytes and macrophages participate critically in the inflammatory activity of various major diseases of atherosclerosis and cancer. For the reduction of inflammation, either monocyte-chemotactic protein (MCP)-1 or CCR2 genetic deletion can result in a profound reduction of inflammation in various disease models [11 - 13]. In a study, Leuschner *et al.* prepared siRNACCR2 lipid nanoformulation for systemic delivery. The results revealed silence of CCR2 gene along with significant reduction of plaque [14]. In coronary artery disease, macrophage-mediated inflammation plays a crucial role. Courties *et al*. studied the efficacy of the siRNA lipid nanoparticles targeting interferon regulatory factor 5 (IRF5). siRNA lipid nanoparticles administration demonstrated infarct healing and attenuated post-myocardial infarction (MI) remodeling [15]. A progressive heart disease, transthyretin (TTR) amyloidosis, causes severe congestive heart failure. Coelho *et al*. used siRNAs encapsulated in lipid nanoparticles that successfully induced transthyretin knockdown in patients with TTR amyloidosis in a phase 1 study [16]. In another study, Patisiran, a lipid nanoparticle formulation of ribonucleic acid interference (RNAi), offered new treatment options for patients with hereditary transthyretin-mediated amyloidosis. With the administration of patisiran, TTR level can be significantly reduced which can improve patient's neuropathy and quality of life [17]. A novel lipid-based nanoformulation of PCSK9 siRNA (inclisiran) showed rapid and durable effects with a single dose in rodents and monkeys. The levels of PCSK9 and LDL were reduced effectively for at least 6 months by using Inclisiran. This displayed a better progress in cardiovascular medicine and was driven by nanotechnology enabled stable delivery of RNA interference therapeutics [18]. Gao *et al*. utilized copper sulfide nanoparticles as a photothermal switch for transient receptor potential vanilloid subfamily 1(TRPV1) signaling to attenuate atherosclerosis. The TRPV1 was conjugated to copper sulfide nanoparticles that induced autophagy in vascular smooth muscle cells and reduced lipid accumulation as well as prevented foam cell formation. On irradiation of the aortic arch of *apoE*$^{-/-}$ mice, there was an increase in local temperature because of the characteristic near-infrared absorption of copper sulfide nanoparticles that generates a strong photoacoustic signal and which opened TRPV1 channels and allowed an influx of calcium ions to activate autophagy [19].

MICRORNA BASED APPLICATIONS

MicroRNA (miRNA) is involved in the normal functioning of eukaryotic cells and function in the heart; dysregulation of miRNA has been associated with the disease. miRNA is used in cardiovascular diseases to know about its expression levels for diagnosis, prognosis or risk stratification [20]. The animal model study is also considered to obtain information about cholesterol metabolism and regulation. Various studies have demonstrated the importance of family members of miR-181during the end-stage heart failure [21, 22]. There has been found an upregulation of miR-181c under different pathological conditions of heart disease, type II diabetes, obesity, and aging [21 - 23]. Overexpression of miR-181c causes oxidative stress, leading to a cardiac-dysfunction [21]. Kent *et al*. developed liposomal nanoparticles for the systemic delivery of the miR-181-sponge construct (specifically designed to include 10 repeated anti-miR-181 binding sequences). To drive the cardio-specific miR-181 miRNA-sponge expression, a cardio-specific α-MHC promoter is cloned into the pEGFP backbone. A study revealed a significant downregulation of the entire miR-181 family (miR-181a, miR-181b, miR-181c, and miR-181d) with the expression of the miR-181-sponge both in *in vitro* and *in vivo* studies; further, these results have been validated through western blot analysis. This approach would be an ideal one; however, if one family member has a detrimental effect within the same organ then miRNA-sponge technology would be appropriate [24]. Antunes *et al.* developed miR-15--5p-poly(isobutylcyanoacrylate)-polysaccharide nanoparticles to evaluate their use as a potential injectable cardio-protective therapy for myocardial infarction. Human coronary artery endothelial cells (hCAECs) cultured with the miR-155-5p loaded nanoparticles illustrated increased content of miR-155-5p and decreased content of BACH1. The silencing of BACH1 within hCAECs gives hope that it will decrease the overall detrimental effects within infarcted hearts which opens a new perspective for therapeutic approaches for cardiovascular diseases [25]. Generally, for the prevention and treatment of CVD, the attention is being paid to lowering circulating LDL cholesterol. In this regard, miRNAs have emerged as an exciting therapeutic target for CVD. At all stages of atherosclerosis, some miRNAs modulate efflux of excess cholesterol from lipid-laden macrophages in the vessel wall to the liver. Nguyen *et al.* developed chitosan nanoparticles for safe delivery of functional miRNA which can effectively alter and reverse cholesterol efflux and transport *in vivo* [26]. When miR33- chitosan nanoparticles were administered to mice, there was observed decreased level of reverse cholesterol transport (RCT) in the plasma, liver and feces. These results suggest that miRNA nanoparticles can be used to target atherosclerotic lesions *in vivo* . Bejerano *et al.* developed hyaluronan-sulfate-Ca^{2+}-miRNA nanoparticles to target cardiac macrophages. After intravenous administration to MI mice, the pro-inflammatory reaction was switched to reparative, reducing hypertrophy, promoting angiogenesis, fibrosis, and cell apoptosis in remote myocardium to prevent heart failure compared to control mice [27]. During a cardiac injury process, mutual cross-talk between miRNAs and ROS exists. To image such type of activity. Yang *et al.* developed crown-like silica@polydopamine-DNA-CeO_2 nanocomposite for detecting and imaging miR-21 and hydrogen peroxide in simulated IR injury in living cells and *in vivo* . In H9C2 rat cardiomyocytes cell line, the miRNA-21 was regulated by H_2O_2 *via* PI3K/AKT signaling pathway. In mimicked condition of heart ischemia-reperfusion injury, H_2O_2 and miRNA-21 were overproduced, suggesting that they are closely related to reperfusion injury [28].

DNA BASED APPLICATIONS

Atherosclerosis is a pathological process of plaque development due to the retention of lipids in the artery wall, which supports the progression of CVD. This hallmark feature gradually leads to stroke and MI [29]. However, the progression of atherosclerosis is slow and symptomatic, hence early detection of the atherosclerotic plaques will benefit the diagnosis of CVD [30]. In this regard, bionanomaterials have been developed as contrast agents to image atherosclerotic plaques. Zhang *et al*. developed DNA-coated PEG-superparamagnetic iron oxide nanoparticles (DNA-SPIONs) as an effective strategy for systemic delivery to atherosclerotic plaques. DNA-SPIONs were administered intravenously to apolipoprotein E knockout (ApoE$^{-/-}$) mice, which enter the macrophages faster and more abundantly using Class A scavenger receptors (SR-A), lipid rafts and traffic inside the cell than that of PEG-SPIONs. Localization of DNA-SPIONs was observed through near-infrared fluorescence imaging in the heart and aorta 30 min post-injection, which gradually climbs to the highest peak at 8h [31]. Perlstein *et al*. used denatured collagen PLGA-coated stents containing plasmid DNA (encoding GFP) for enhancement of gene transfer. The study conducted on pig coronary artery with denatured collagen incorporated plasmid DNA-stent coating illustrated increased level of gene expression in the arterial smooth muscle cell cytoskeleton due to integrin-related mechanisms compared to without DNA-coated stents [32].

CONCLUDING REMARKS

The focus of clinical translation for the RNA interference is on gene silencing and appropriate dosing requirement in the course of treatments. In recent years, it has become increasingly important to consider the degradability of siRNA delivery materials and their potential for immune stimulation. The future work needs to focus on the potency of the nanovehicle and its clinical translation towards transient RNA interference therapy.

CONSENT FOR PUBLICATION

Not Applicable.

CONFLICT OF INTEREST

The author confirms that this chapter contents have no conflict of interest.

ACKNOWLEDGEMENT

FD gratefully acknowledges Dept. of Science and Technology, Govt. of India, for the financial grant [SR/WOS-A/LS-448/2017(G)] in the form of women scientist fellowship (WOS-A).

REFERENCES

[1]   Whitehead KA, Langer R, Anderson DG. Knocking down barriers: advances in siRNA delivery. Nat Rev Drug Discov 2009; 8(2): 129-38.
[http://dx.doi.org/10.1038/nrd2742] [PMID: 19180106]

[2]   Frank-Kamenetsky M, Grefhorst A, Anderson NN, *et al.* Therapeutic RNAi targeting PCSK9 acutely lowers plasma cholesterol in rodents and LDL cholesterol in nonhuman primates. Proc Natl Acad Sci USA 2008; 105(33): 11915-20.
[http://dx.doi.org/10.1073/pnas.0805434105] [PMID: 18695239]

[3]   Song E, Lee SK, Wang J, *et al.* RNA interference targeting Fas protects mice from fulminant hepatitis. Nat Med 2003; 9(3): 347-51.
[http://dx.doi.org/10.1038/nm828] [PMID: 12579197]

[4]   Sato Y, Murase K, Kato J, *et al.* Resolution of liver cirrhosis using vitamin A-coupled liposomes to deliver siRNA against a collagen-specific chaperone. Nat Biotechnol 2008; 26(4): 431-42.
[http://dx.doi.org/10.1038/nbt1396] [PMID: 18376398]

[5]   Takeshita F, Minakuchi Y, Nagahara S, *et al.* Efficient delivery of small interfering RNA to bone-metastatic tumors by using atelocollagen *in vivo* . Proc Natl Acad Sci USA 2005; 102(34): 12177-82.
[http://dx.doi.org/10.1073/pnas.0501753102] [PMID: 16091473]

[6]   Halder J, Kamat AA, Landen CN Jr, *et al.* Focal adhesion kinase targeting using *in vivo* short interfering RNA delivery in neutral liposomes for ovarian carcinoma therapy. Clin Cancer Res 2006; 12(16): 4916-24.
[http://dx.doi.org/10.1158/1078-0432.CCR-06-0021] [PMID: 16914580]

[7]   Aouadi M, Tesz GJ, Nicoloro SM, *et al.* Orally delivered siRNA targeting macrophage Map4k4 suppresses systemic inflammation. Nature 2009; 458(7242): 1180-4.
[http://dx.doi.org/10.1038/nature07774] [PMID: 19407801]

[8]   Blow N. Small RNAs: delivering the future. Nature 2007; 450(7172): 1117-20.
[http://dx.doi.org/10.1038/4501117a] [PMID: 18075597]

[9]   Li JM, Newburger PE, Gounis MJ, Dargon P, Zhang X, Messina LM. Local arterial nanoparticle delivery of siRNA for NOX2 knockdown to prevent restenosis in an atherosclerotic rat model. Gene Ther 2010; 17(10): 1279-87.
[http://dx.doi.org/10.1038/gt.2010.69] [PMID: 20485380]

[10]   Hossfeld S, Nolte A, Hartmann H, *et al.* Bioactive coronary stent coating based on layer-by-layer technology for siRNA release. Acta Biomater 2013; 9(5): 6741-52.
[http://dx.doi.org/10.1016/j.actbio.2013.01.013] [PMID: 23333865]

[11]   Abdi R, Means TK, Ito T, *et al.* Differential role of CCR2 in islet and heart allograft rejection: tissue specificity of chemokine/chemokine receptor function *in vivo* . J Immunol 2004; 172(2): 767-75.
[http://dx.doi.org/10.4049/jimmunol.172.2.767] [PMID: 14707046]

[12]   Boring L, Gosling J, Cleary M, Charo IF. Decreased lesion formation in CCR2-/- mice reveals a role for chemokines in the initiation of atherosclerosis. Nature 1998; 394(6696): 894-7.
[http://dx.doi.org/10.1038/29788] [PMID: 9732872]

[13]   Kaikita K, Hayasaki T, Okuma T, Kuziel WA, Ogawa H, Takeya M. Targeted deletion of CC chemokine receptor 2 attenuates left ventricular remodeling after experimental myocardial infarction. Am J Pathol 2004; 165(2): 439-47.
[http://dx.doi.org/10.1016/S0002-9440(10)63309-3] [PMID: 15277218]

[14]   Leuschner F, Dutta P, Gorbatov R, *et al.* Therapeutic siRNA silencing in inflammatory monocytes in mice. Nat Biotechnol 2011; 29(11): 1005-10.
[http://dx.doi.org/10.1038/nbt.1989] [PMID: 21983520]

[15]   Courties G, Heidt T, Sebas M, *et al. In vivo* silencing of the transcription factor IRF5 reprograms the macrophage phenotype and improves infarct healing. J Am Coll Cardiol 2014; 63(15): 1556-66.

[http://dx.doi.org/10.1016/j.jacc.2013.11.023] [PMID: 24361318]

[16] Coelho T, Adams D, Silva A, *et al.* Safety and efficacy of RNAi therapy for transthyretin amyloidosis. N Engl J Med 2013; 369(9): 819-29.
[http://dx.doi.org/10.1056/NEJMoa1208760] [PMID: 23984729]

[17] Yang J. Patisiran for the treatment of hereditary transthyretin-mediated amyloidosis. Expert Rev Clin Pharmacol 2019; 12(2): 95-9.
[http://dx.doi.org/10.1080/17512433.2019.1567326] [PMID: 30644768]

[18] Whitehead KA, Dorkin JR, Vegas AJ, *et al.* Degradable lipid nanoparticles with predictable *in vivo* siRNA delivery activity. Nat Commun 2014; 5(4277): 4277.
[http://dx.doi.org/10.1038/ncomms5277] [PMID: 24969323]

[19] Gao W, Sun Y, Cai M, *et al.* Copper sulfide nanoparticles as a photothermal switch for TRPV1 signaling to attenuate atherosclerosis. Nat Commun 2018; 9(1): 231.
[http://dx.doi.org/10.1038/s41467-017-02657-z] [PMID: 29335450]

[20] Keller A, Rounge T, Backes C, *et al.* Sources to variability in circulating human miRNA signatures. RNA Biol 2017; 14(12): 1791-8.
[http://dx.doi.org/10.1080/15476286.2017.1367888] [PMID: 28820329]

[21] Das S, Bedja D, Campbell N, *et al.* miR-181c regulates the mitochondrial genome, bioenergetics, and propensity for heart failure *in vivo* . PLoS One 2014; 9(5): e96820.
[http://dx.doi.org/10.1371/journal.pone.0096820] [PMID: 24810628]

[22] Zhu X, Wang H, Liu F, *et al.* Identification of micro-RNA networks in end-stage heart failure because of dilated cardiomyopathy. J Cell Mol Med 2013; 17(9): 1173-87.
[http://dx.doi.org/10.1111/jcmm.12096] [PMID: 23998897]

[23] Das S, Kohr M, Dunkerly-Eyring B, *et al.* Divergent effects of miR-181 family members on myocardial function through protective cytosolic and detrimental mitochondrial microRNA targets. J Am Heart Assoc 2017; 6(3): e004694.
[http://dx.doi.org/10.1161/JAHA.116.004694] [PMID: 28242633]

[24] Kent OA, Steenbergen C, Das S. *In vivo* nanovector delivery of a heart-specific microrna-sponge. J Vis Exp 2018; 136(136): e57845.
[http://dx.doi.org/10.3791/57845] [PMID: 29985373]

[25] Antunes JC, Benarroch L, Moraes FC, *et al.* Core-shell polymer-based nanoparticles deliver mir-15--5p to endothelial cells. Mol Ther Nucleic Acids 2019; 17: 210-22.
[http://dx.doi.org/10.1016/j.omtn.2019.05.016] [PMID: 31265949]

[26] Nguyen MA, Wyatt H, Susser L, *et al.* Delivery of micrornas by chitosan nanoparticles to functionally alter macrophage cholesterol efflux *in vitro* and *in vivo* . ACS Nano 2019; 13(6): 6491-505.
[http://dx.doi.org/10.1021/acsnano.8b09679] [PMID: 31125197]

[27] Bejerano T, Etzion S, Elyagon S, Etzion Y, Cohen S. Nanoparticle delivery of mirna-21 mimic to cardiac macrophages improves myocardial remodeling after myocardial infarction. Nano Lett 2018; 18(9): 5885-91.
[http://dx.doi.org/10.1021/acs.nanolett.8b02578] [PMID: 30141949]

[28] Yang L, Ren Y, Pan W, *et al.* Fluorescent nanocomposite for visualizing cross-talk between microRNA-21 and hydrogen peroxide in ischemia-Reperfusion Injury in Live Cells and *in vivo* . Anal Chem 2016; 88(23): 11886-91.
[http://dx.doi.org/10.1021/acs.analchem.6b03701] [PMID: 27804287]

[29] Hansson GK, Hermansson A. The immune system in atherosclerosis. Nat Immunol 2011; 12(3): 204-12.
[http://dx.doi.org/10.1038/ni.2001] [PMID: 21321594]

[30] Mulder WJM, Jaffer FA, Fayad ZA, Nahrendorf M. Imaging and nanomedicine in inflammatory atherosclerosis. Sci Transl Med 2014; 6(239): 239sr1.

[http://dx.doi.org/10.1126/scitranslmed.3005101] [PMID: 24898749]

[31]   Zhang L, Tian XY, Chan CKW, *et al.* Promoting the delivery of nanoparticles to atherosclerotic plaques by DNA Coating. ACS Appl Mater Interfaces 2019; 11(15): 13888-904.
[http://dx.doi.org/10.1021/acsami.8b17928] [PMID: 30516979]

[32]   Perlstein I, Connolly JM, Cui X, *et al.* DNA delivery from an intravascular stent with a denatured collagen-polylactic-polyglycolic acid-controlled release coating: mechanisms of enhanced transfection. Gene Ther 2003; 10(17): 1420-8.
[http://dx.doi.org/10.1038/sj.gt.3302043] [PMID: 12900756]

CHAPTER 8

Ethics and Regulations for Cardiovascular Diseases

Ajit Kumar Behura[1,*], **Sarita Kar**[1] and **Fahima Dilnawaz**[2,*]

[1] *Department of Humanities and Social Sciences, Indian Institute of Technology (ISM) Dhandbad, Dhandbad-826004, Jharkhand, India*

[2] *Laboratory of Nanomedicine, Institute of Life Sciences, Nalco Square, Chandrasekharpur, Bhubaneswar-751023, Odisha, India*

Abstract: Ethics deals with human values and conduct, with respect to right and wrong in certain motives. The rapid development of therapeutics has raised a number of ethical issues pertaining to philosophical, legal, religious and moral beliefs. With the advancement of science, inclusion of ethical values is of absolute necessity in different aspects of clinical practice. The introduction of nanotechnology has helped in fighting many complex illnesses, including cardiovascular diseases. Nanotechnology may provide a solution for better prognoses and a reduced side effect. In this regard, cardiovascular therapeutic involvement needs a testimony with respect to societal benefits for developing a code of ethics.

Keywords: Autonomy, Beneficence, Ethics, Morality.

INTRODUCTION

Cardiovascular diseases (CVDs) are a group of disorders related to the heart and blood vessels. CVDs have become one of the common causes of death due to unhealthy diet, physical inactivity, alcohol and tobacco use, leading to 31% of deaths worldwide [1]. Apart from that, coping up with urbanization, intense involvement in industrialized work and related lifestyle changes have been associated with high blood pressure, raised blood lipids, high blood glucose levels leading to overweight and obesity, and an increased risk of developing a heart stroke, heart failure and related complications. The related severe complications of CVDs are a very frequent reason for the hospitalization of patients. However, modern treatments have intensely improved the quality of life of cases with

---

[*] **Corresponding authors Fahima Dilnawaz & Dr Ajit Kumar Behura:** Laboratory of Nanomedicine. Institute of Life Sciences, Nalco Square. Bhubaneswar-751023, India. Department of, Humanities and Social Sciences, Indian Institute of Technology (ISM) Dhandbad, Dhandbad-826004, Jharkhand, India; Tel: +91-674 – 2304341, 2304283, Fax: 91-674-2300728; E-mail: fahimadilnawaz@gmail.com and Tel:+91-326-2235499, Fax: + 91-326- 2296563; E-mail: ajitbehura@gmail.com

hypertension, valvular heart disease, coronary artery disease, and mild heart failure.

Patients with chronic CVD problems, such as congestive heart failure, need continued medical support with the intervention of expensive medical care for their long-term survival [2]. Beyond medication, technology has advanced with the supply of medical devices to improve symptom burden and prolong the patients' survival. The CVDs therapeutic activity has broadened from being principally curative to being preventive [3, 4]. The identification of various factors responsible for CVD diseases is required to predict the risk associated with CVD diseases and implement diagnostic methods for early detection and prevention. In clinical research trials, many invasive cardiologists are involved. Frequently, invasive cardiologists usually perform dual roles as a clinical researcher as well as a treating clinician. Often this is programmed by the industry to evaluate their products and enroll patients in their trials for which they provide a variety of incentives and financial aids to the clinical researchers. While doing this activity, clinicians have to remember all the time that their first commitment is towards their patient. However, during the course of treatment, if the clinician gets to know that there is another avenue for the patient, then the clinician-researcher should withdraw the subject (enrolled patient) from the research trial supporting subject's best interest. For doing this kind of dual-mode research and treatment, the patients must be fully informed. Further, if critically ill patients are involved, then great caution should be taken into account [5].

Cardiovascular diseases are multivarious in nature; therefore, several guidelines have been established for their prevention in clinical practice while taking into the account their scientific understanding. In the case of symptomatic treatment, the drugs are advised by the clinicians for purely preventive purposes, whereas with the advancement of the disease, sometimes the intervention of specific medical devices pertaining to the ailment is needed. This may pose some kind of ethical dilemma. In that case, the cost-effectiveness of the treatment for the patient can somehow increase the pressure on the medical community. Therefore, the medical fraternity should take into consideration the financial burden while evaluating the potential benefit as well as the long-term consequence of the therapeutic interventions. While dealing with the increased number of cardiac-related medical cases, complex societal bound medical care and patient's budgetary restrictions sometimes remainone of the major decisive factors. In this case, preventive medicine should remain as one of the choices in clinical practice. The principal values of medical ethics and their application in different aspects of secondary and primary CVDs prevention are discussed in the following section.Since the earliest recorded history of medicine, "Codes of medical ethics" have existed. With time, the medical practice has evolved and modified. The American Medical

Association (AMA) first adopted a general code of ethics in 1847 and revised it most recently in 1997 [6]. In medicine, "medical ethics" is the study of moral values and judgements. The medical fraternity treating CVDs should set the Code of Ethics in their clinical practice and should have certain ethical obligations to their patients, as well as to the community and world at large. The clinicians being a member of the medical profession must respect, recognize, and adhere to these obligations [7, 8]. The main principles that are laid down in "Code of Ethics" are mentioned below: (i) Beneficence; actions in the best interests of patients (ii) Primum non nocere: first of all, do no harm to patients (iii) Autonomy; right of the patients to choose or refuse their treatment (iv) Informed consent; truthfulness and honesty and (v) Justice; fairness in the distribution of health resources [9, 10].

GENERAL ETHICAL IMPLICATIONS

Actions in the best interests of patients (Beneficence): (i) The ethical principle of 'beneficence' states that the clinicians should make an attempt for the improvement of patient's well-being with a provision of maximal clinical benefits while minimizing clinical harms. (ii) First, do no harm (primum non nocere; non-maleficence): The principle of 'non-maleficence' urges the clinicians not to cause any intentional harm for incurring greater benefits; rather, they should respect patients' clinical concerns. (iii) In the case of autonomy, the patient has the absolute right to choose or refuse their treatment and can make a rational uninfluenced decision whether to get treated under a particular clinician or not. (iv) truthfulness and honesty (informed consent). The principle of informed consent is applicable to the patients, where the patient is fully informed regarding the understandability of the potential benefits and risks of their choice of treatment, whereas an uninformed person can be at risk of mistakenly making a choice of not knowing the facts. (v) fairness in the distribution of health resources (justice). In this case, the clinicians are the best advocate to suggest what type of treatment is necessary for the patient, and accordingly take decision as to what kind of treatment should be given to whom after looking at the availability of the health resources. These principles can be applied when the benefits and risks for interventions are clear, but in uncertainty, it can be challenging. In this regard, patient-centered approach can be applied to involve (vi) the ethical principle 'respect for persons' in which the clinicians are required to respect the autonomy of patients and to function as a chaperone in accordance with patients' values, beliefs and preferences.

CONSENT FOR PUBLICATION

Not Applicable.

CONFLICT OF INTEREST

The author confirms that this chapter contents have no conflict of interest.

ACKNOWLEDGEMENT

FD gratefully acknowledges Dept. of Science and Technology, Govt. of India, for the financial grant [SR/WOS-A/LS-448/2017(G)] in the form of women scientist fellowship (WOS-A).

REFERENCES

[1]   https://www.who.int/health-topics/cardiovascular-diseases

[2]   https://www.cdc.gov/heartdisease/facts.htm

[3]   https://www.webmd.com/heart-disease/guide/diseases-cardiovascular#1

[4]   Velagaleti RS, Pencina MJ, Murabito JM, *et al.* Long-term trends in the incidence of heart failure after myocardial infarction. Circulation 2008; 118(20): 2057-62.
       [http://dx.doi.org/10.1161/CIRCULATIONAHA.108.784215] [PMID: 18955667]

[5]   Cameron AAC, Laskey WK, Sheldon WC. Society for Cardiovascular Angiography and Interventions (SCAI) ad hoc task force on ethics in invasive and interventional cardiology. Ethical issues for invasive cardiologists: Society for cardiovascular angiography and interventions. Catheter Cardiovasc Interv 2004; 61(2): 157-62.
       [http://dx.doi.org/10.1002/ccd.10800] [PMID: 14755804]

[6]   Baker R, Caplan A, Emanuel LL, Latham SR. Crisis, ethics, and the american medical association 1847 and 1997. JAMA 1997; 278(2): 163-4.
       [http://dx.doi.org/10.1001/jama.1997.03550020095046] [PMID: 9214535]

[7]   Frye RL, Simari RD, Gersh BJ, *et al.* Ethical issues in cardiovascular research involving humans. Circulation 2009; 120(21): 2113-21.
       [http://dx.doi.org/10.1161/CIRCULATIONAHA.107.752766] [PMID: 19933950]

[8]   Gillon R. Medical ethics: four principles plus attention to scope. BMJ 1994; 309(6948): 184-8.
       [http://dx.doi.org/10.1136/bmj.309.6948.184] [PMID: 8044100]

[9]   https://www.acc.org/about-acc/our-bylaws-and-code-of-ethics/code-of-ethics

[10]   Beauchamp TL, Childress JF. Principles of Biomedical Ethics. Oxford Univ Press 2013; pp. 0-480.

CHAPTER 9

Biomaterials for Cardiac Regeneration

Nazia Hassan[1], Pooja Jain[1], Salma Firdaus[1] and Zeenat Iqbal[1,*]

[1] *Department of Pharmaceutics, School of Pharmaceutical Education and Research (SPER), Jamia Hamdard, New Delhi-110062, India*

Abstract: Globally, cardiovascular disease is one of the predominant clinical conditions, which accounts for about 50% of human mortality and morbidity. No doubt pharmacological and surgical interventions have dramatically improved the quality of life of patients with cardiovascular diseases. However, the demand for new therapeutic interventions as well as regenerative strategies is currently increasing. Biomaterials, both natural and synthetic, have exhibited great potential in cardiac regenerative therapy. Therefore, the development of biomaterials based extracellular matrix, grafts or stents, *etc.* would be highly beneficial for supporting the natural function and physiology of heart tissues.

Keywords: Biohybrid vascular grafts, Bioresorbable stents, Bioceramics, Cardiac patches, Extracellular matrix, Hydrogels, Implants, Scaffolds.

INTRODUCTION

Heart is one of the major organs of the human body which starts functioning in the first three weeks of gestation. Any disease or condition either relating to or acting on the heart is medically termed as 'Cardiac'. Normally, the human heart pumps approx. 175–224 millionliters of blood throughout the body with the help of a unique subset of cells, cardiomyocytes, present in the heart muscle (myocardium). These cells are intimately connected to one another through gap junctions and produce a synchronous contractile response to electrical stimulations. The human heart is composed of a diverse cellular structure, mainly cardiomyocytes (contractile elements), smooth muscle cells, fibroblasts, blood vessels, nerves and the extracellular matrix (ECM) components (collagen). Cardiomyocytes normally have the limited ability to proliferate (average proliferation rate < 1% annually). Any impairment or disability of the tissues and

* **Corresponding author Zeenat Iqbal:** Department of Pharmaceutics, School of Pharmaceutical Education and Research (SPER), Jamia Hamdard, New Delhi-110062, India; E-mail: zeenatiqbal@jamiahamdard.ac.in

Fahima Dilnawaz and Zeenat Iqbal (Eds.)

cells may lead to irreversible heart damage such as ischemic/ hypertensive/ valvular heart disease, myocardial infarction, *etc.*, which can subsequently lead to a condition of heart failure (impairment of blood pumping efficiency) [1, 2].

Therefore, novel treatment approaches are urgently needed to control and regulate the rampant prevalence of cardiac diseases. Conventional treatment modalities such as medications, surgical interventions (bypass grafts, valvular change, stenting, *etc.*) are marred with various challenges. Further, in acute cases, heart transplants are highly unlikely due to the chronic shortage of human tissue donors. In order to expand the patient care options, alternative therapies based on biomaterials are utilized for repairing, reconstructing or regenerating damaged/impaired heart tissues or cells [3 - 7]. Biomaterials (BM), in general, can be defined as foreign, non-drug material that is accepted to be used inside the body for the purpose of enhancement of tissue/organ functions, as well as to repair the damaged/impaired organ(s) in a variety of clinical conditions. BMs can either be synthetic or natural and are mostly biocompatible in nature so that they can have safe interaction with the biological system (body fluids, soft tissues, *etc.*). The term biocompatibility generally signifies its patient compliance, mechanical as well as biological properties in varied processes of implantation, cardiovascular repair/regeneration, tissue replacement, *etc.* The BM should possess the properties of durability, strength, flexibility and minimum ability to elicit any adverse reactions. They are generally integrated into a device or can be used on their own for replacement purposes in order to mimic the characteristics of the required heart tissue. Whereas, their biological properties are anti-thrombogenicity, hemostasis, endothelialization, non-calcification, non-immunogenicity, non-toxicity and inertness [8, 9]. Historically, the use of BMs for medicinal purposes is a widely evolving global concept. Ancient Phoenicians have exploited, for dental work, gold wires like BM to hold artificial teeth with the real ones [1]. Further, in the era of the 19th century, artificial bone plates were introduced to help to stabilize bone fracture and to facilitate the healing process. Currently, the use of BMs has been extended to the development of cardiovascular components such as heart valves, blood vessels, scaffolds, gauges, *etc.*, thereby marking their efficiency in the field of cardiac tissue repair and regeneration [10]. The chapter explores the future prospects in terms of biomaterials-based regenerative medicines and also highlights the bioethical aspects of safety, regulatory and ethical issues.

TYPES OF BIOMATERIALS

Biomaterials can be broadly classified into four main categories, depending upon the nature of the source as presented below:

Natural

These are mainly those BMs which are derived from plant or animal sources such as collagen, alginate, coral, keratin, cellulose, *etc.* Naturally derived BMs can also be obtained from humans, either as auto-graft, allograft or iso-graft. They can be either used on their own or in conjugation with a device. Most often, natural derived BMs are basically used for healing purposes rather than replacement therapy [9 - 11]. Natural BMs could be either (i) Xenogenic (animal-derived), which can be used for developing pericardium, collagen patch, or for septal defect repair [12]. (ii) Allogenic (same-species donor), which can be employed for creating pericardium, fibro serous sac surrounding the mammalian heart, for reconstruction, valve repair and aortic root enlargement [13] or (iii) Autogenic (same individual), wherein the BMs can be used for valve replacement [13, 14].

Metal-based Biomaterials

Metals are the most widely used material for BMs that can be either of pure metals or alloys. Due to various intrinsic properties of metals such as tensile strength, relative inertness, malleability and ductility, and higher resistance to mechanical wear, they are used to construct a wide array of parts such as wires, screws, stents, bone plates, prosthetic limbs, and joint replacement, among others. The most commonly used metals are stainless steel, titanium, gold and silver which are mostly non-reactive and biocompatible in nature. Alloys such as titanium and cobalt are also used. However, these metal-derived BMs have the drawback of corrosion, which limits their use for long-term therapy [9 - 11]. A few common examples of metal BMs and their applications are presented below: (i) Metals stents for the purpose of opening lumen in obstructed heart vessels. The classic examples are titanium and stainless steel; however, owing to their comparative greater strength, the present stent design also utilizes cobalt-chromium, platinum-chromium and nickel-titanium alloys [15 - 17]. (ii) to minimize the risk of blood clot formation, mechanical replacement of heart valves using stainless steel or titanium is utilized [18, 19].

Ceramics-based Biomaterials

Ceramic biomaterials or bioceramics are refractory polycrystalline compounds that are known to be widely used in dentistry over very long periods. Usually, they are inorganic, highly inert, hard, brittle, and compressive with good electric and thermal insulation strength. Additionally, the aesthetic appearance of bioceramics highly compliments the aforementioned attributes, making them a better choice for dentistry applications. However, drawbacks like poor fracture, toughness and biocompatibility issue limit the incorporation of bioceramics in cardiac-related treatments. The most common examples of bioceramics are aluminium oxide, calcium phosphates, and hydroxyapatite carbon [20, 21]. Bioceramics are particularly used in restorative material dental inlays, onlays, veneers, crowns/bridges and dentures [22] and are also exploited for making orthopedics implants, such as the femoral head, bone screws and plates [20].

Polymer-based Biomaterials

They can be both natural as well as synthetically derived. They are one of the most widely used materials for the development of BMs. They are used in the form of medical adhesives, sealants and coatings for replacement and restorative purposes. The main disadvantage associated with polymers is their relatively low strength and increased chances of degradation and deformation with time [9 - 11]. Polymers are modified (engrafted with pharmaceuticals, growth factors, *etc.*) for drug delivery and gene therapy [23 - 25]. Polyurethanes (PUs), also known as reaction polymers, are widely exploited for valve repair therapy owing to their strength, elasticity, transparency, infection resistance and easy handling [26, 27]. Various *in vitro* investigations have used thermoplastic PU for cardiac stem cell therapy [28, 29].

Composites-based Biomaterials

In this type, both natural and synthetic materials are used for producing composite materials in order to multiply their advantages and limit the unwanted effects such as limited durability, a higher chance of thrombosis, *etc.* The composite BMs are fortified with superior attributes of functionality, strength, durability, biocompatibility, but they lack robustness. Composites can be prepared by blending (only physical combination), coating *via* submersion or spraying, copolymerizing (modification of polymer structure into monomers of multiple blocks), followed by polymerization and multilayering or sandwiching of materials *via* mechanical fixation. The major disadvantage of composites is their low elastic modulus [30 - 34]. A few popular examples of composites include (i) Dental filling, (ii) Prosthetic limbs, owing to their dual advantage of being light weight and high overall strength, (iii) Polymeric material based bioprosthetic valves can be incorporated for overcoming the lack of tissue strength [35].

APPLICATION OF BIOMATERIALS

The applications of BMs have increased significantly in therapy and diagnostics. Earlier, the use of BMs was restricted to the restorative or supportive function, as in the dental implants, bone plates, *etc.* Since the concept of biocompatibility was not well known, any material which was suitably tolerated by the body was used. As science and technology progressed, BMs were increasingly used as soft tissue replacements. A few of the vastly evolved examples of BMs application [36, 37] are as follows:

Medical Implants

These are used to replace diseased or damaged tissues or organs for restoring the function of the organ/tissue. These include heart valves, dental implants, hip joints and parts of the kidney and liver. These medical implants can also be used for the replacement of tendons and ligaments.

Aiding in the Healing of Human Tissues

Besides tissue repair and regeneration, the BMs also assist either in the healing process or speed it up by virtue of providing additional support. Examples of BMs used for enhanced healing are sutures, screws, bone plates, clips, staples for wound closing, dissolvable dressing, *etc*. Such BMs do not actively participate in the healing process itself but aid in the process.

Regeneration of Damaged Tissues

Similar to the above-mentioned function, the BMs used in this case are employed in conjugation with natural materials such as cells and other bioactive molecules. These BMs are responsible for providing support (scaffolding), whereas the bioactive elements help in the regeneration process for bone regenerating hydrogels.

Improve the Function or Correct Functional Abnormalities

This is one of the most exploited traditional uses of BMs. The function of an organ/tissue can be improved by providing support/aid by using biomaterial in conjugation with a device or/and equipment. Examples of such uses are the cardiac pacemaker, intra-ocular lens, *etc*.

Correct Cosmetic Problems

BMs are widely used in the cosmetic industry, either for purposes such as chin reshaping, mastectomy augmentation, or for more aesthetic purposes such as face lifts, lip fillers, *etc*.

Aid in Detection and Treatment

Biosensors and molecular probes are often used in the medical field to detect and combat various diseases such as cancer, diabetes, *etc*. These devices can circumvent the problem of biological barriers giving us better imaging and detection of diseases such as cancer. Apart from this, biosensors can be lifesaving in patients with diabetes, where these can be used to detect the blood glucose levels. BM can also be employed in the treatment with the use of devices such as catheters and probes.

Drug Delivery System

BMs are increasingly being used for targeted drug delivery of drug molecules. Various polymers (natural and synthetic) are used to modify or improve the targeted drug delivery to a diseased organ.

Biomaterial-based Cardiac Regeneration Strategies

BMs are extensively used in cardiac regenerative, restorative and replacement therapy. BMs are used in cardiac therapy as heart pacemakers, regenerative cell therapy, and artificial heart valves [36 - 38]. The selection of biomaterials is based on a variety of parameters; however, the main points that need to be considered are the properties of the BMs and the purpose of their use. From a safety perspective, the characteristic of BMs is of immense importance. The BMs used should be inert, non-toxic and non-reactive with the body tissue and fluid, and most importantly, should not incite any immunological reaction in the body [7 - 11]. As the property of biocompatibility has become prominent, more studies have been done, and based on them, the selection of BMs is as follows:

Biomaterial Design Implication

Various attributes involved in the design of BMs can be broadly classified into two groups, namely mechanical and biological, depending upon their selection and involvement in diverse clinical conditions [9 - 11].

Mechanical Attributes

These mainly encompass durability, stability and flexibility of BMs to maintain natural cardiac rhythm (contraction and relaxation), blood flow, vessel walls pressure, *etc.*, during or after the process of implantation, cardiovascular repair/regeneration and tissue replacement.

Biological Properties

These involve the ability of BMs to either counter or lower adverse effects such as thrombosis, stenosis, haemostasis, endothelialisation, calcification, immunogenicity and toxicity during or after the process of implantation, cardiovascular repair/regeneration and tissue replacement. Apart from the aforementioned attributes, the other factors involved in design of BMs are as follows:

Sterilizability

Since the BMs and conjugated devices are used inside the body, they should be highly sterilizable. These materials should be able to withstand different sterilization conditions such as high temperature, pressure, pH changes, *etc*.

Ease of Manufacturing

BMs are used in a variety of forms, such as gels, fibers, micro-beads to solid shapes like plates, wires, screws, *etc*. A large variety of BMs can be used easily by the manufacturer for different devices and parts.

Physical Properties

Properties such as mechanical strength, elasticity, ductility, malleability, resistance to wear, toughness and hardness, are the deciding factor while selecting BM for various purposes. For example, a BM with a low elastic modulus cannot be used in joint replacement.

Availability of Raw Material and Affordability of Final Product

In order to keep the cost of BMs and its related products reasonable and affordable, it is essential that the raw materials should be easily available. The scarcity of raw material for BM will directly affect the cost of the end product.

Extracellular Matrix as a Biomaterial and its Role in Cardiac Development and Regeneration

Extracellular matrix (ECM) is an important constituent of the human body since the stage of embryogenesis and it provides significant biophysical and chemical components to the growing embryo. Any impairment in the ECM can result in severe defects or embryo death. The role of ECM is to influence every essential cell behavior such as tissue morphogenesis, cardiac development, *etc*. Henceforth, it is critical to evaluate and understand the role of ECM in prevalent pathological conditions such as cardiac repair and regeneration and use it as BM [39, 40]. ECM plays a major role in cardiac repair and regeneration. Any changes or mutation in ECM can lead to a variety of cardiac conditions such as congenital heart defects, cardiovascular diseases, *etc*. At present, the conventional treatment for both cardiovascular and heart diseases is inadequate with various clinical challenges; predominantly, the failure to restore normal functions of the affected tissue following post-surgical process. Such therapies are often palliative in nature and the process for tissue reconstruction is involved with the use of synthetic patches, mechanical valves, *etc*. Moreover, conventional therapeutics may slow down the progression of heart failure but they cannot restore the contractile heart functions; further, the use of synthetic material (patches, valves, *etc.*) may hamper the process of cardiac development. In many cases, cardiac transplant is quintessential for patient's survival; however, the involvement of an organ donor is scarce and which may result in unnecessary complications, most commonly, transfer of infection leading to treatment failure and even death. Therefore, there is an intense demand to develop novel treatment options for cardiac patients. ECM is a naturally derived cardiac matrix which needs to be exploited as a substrate for, *in-vitro* expansion or differentiation of cardiac cells and stem cells toward the cardiomyocyte lineage, as a scaffold or cardiac ECM patch in whole heart engineering (a newer approach in which the heart is decellularized) that can either be seeded with cardiomyocytes or stem cells, and used as an injectable cardiac ECM (where the decellularized ECM is converted to solubilized form) which can be directly injected into the myocardial wall. The aforementioned approaches are promising in producing the anticipated novel effects; further, suitable optimization is required for clinical applications [3, 11, 39, 40]. The rapid progression of fibroblast ECM as BM for cardiac regeneration has gained newer insights into normal cardiac development as well as clinical conditions. Various studies have targeted fibroblasts and evaluated their role in the production of ECM as a dynamic therapeutic approach against cardiovascular diseases.

Biomaterials-Based Cardiac Regenerative Medicines: Future Approach

As discussed above, the concept of biomaterials-based regenerative medicines for cardiac repair and development is an evolving, interdisciplinary therapeutic and research approach. These are often associated with tissue engineering, which facilitates clinically effective and reliable solutions for cardiac transplant, scarcity of organ donor and impairment effects of prosthetics (synthetic or biological) used in cardiac repair and replacement. The clinical features of cardiac diseases vary in patients; therefore, it provides an option to design materials, therapeutic and surgical approaches for transplantation and replacement therapies to restore and balance normal tissue physiology and functions. New imaging and diagnostic tools of biological origin, such as ECM derived scaffolds, injectable hydrogels, cardiac patches, bioresorbable stents and vascular grafts (Fig. **1**), are carefully tailored, optimized and characterized to deal with disease pathology, patients' anatomy and physiology in cardiac repair, replacement and regenerative approaches.

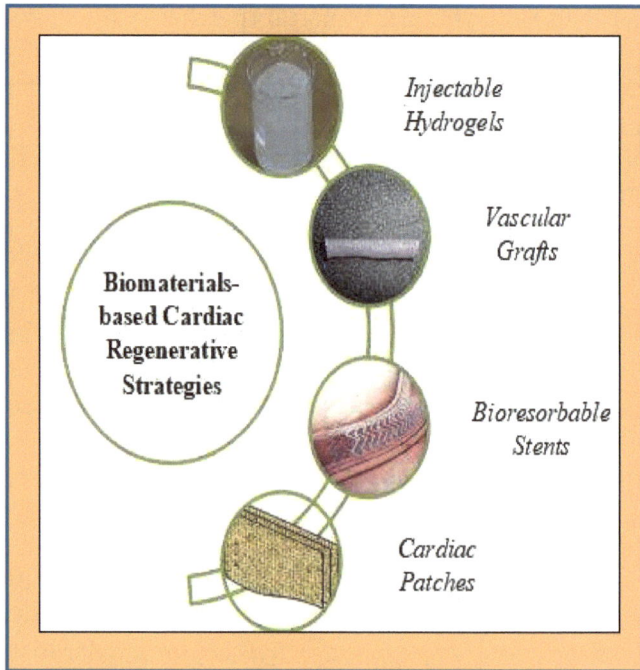

Fig. (1).   Biomaterials-Based Cardiac Regenerative Strategies: Surgical (bioresorbable stents) and Intracoronary (injectable hydrogels, vascular grafts, cardiac patches).

Such devices are designed and fabricated to counter the unmet challenges associated with cardiovascular diseases (myocardial infarction, heart failure, ischemic heart disease, *etc.*, valvular and congenital heart diseases). In all the aforementioned conditions, cardiac cells and tissues are most often represented by delayed response, inability, very low self-regeneration and reperfusion (restoration of blood flow post-ischemic heart diseases) condition. The infarcted regions of cardiac vessels undergo necrosis due to occlusion by thrombus formation. The occurrence of such types of conditions is responsible for a variety of cardiac diseases, making them one of the leading causes of global mortality and morbidity [3, 11, 36 - 38].

REGENERATIVE MEDICINES

Stem cells (embryonic stem cells, mesenchymal stem cells), adipose tissue, and endothelial progenitor cells (peripheral blood, cardiac progenitors) are basically used to restore tissues or organs' impaired functions either by employing surgical or intracoronary approach [41 - 42]. The most widely exploited examples of regenerative biomaterials are presented below:

Injectable Hydrogels

Hybrid hydrogel injections are one of the most widely used techniques for inducing remodeling and substitution of cardiac ECM post-infarction. These hydrogels, after administration, repair and regenerate the myocardial infarctions, subsequently resulting in an improved quality of life of patients. Up till now, various hydrogels designed and fabricated for cardiac tissue regeneration are injected *via* the transcatheter process. Numerous clinical studies have illustrated the use of hydrogels for maintenance and improvement of cardiac functional parameters either alone or in combination with cells as well as growth factors [43 - 44] (Table **1**).

Table 1. Biomaterials-based cardiac regenerative strategies; some of the formulations have entered clinical trials.

Types	Features	References
Alginate hydrogel	Permanent prosthetic scaffold, follows intracoronary infusion, increases scar thickness and ECM concentration, reduces vessel wall stress and enlargement	[45]
Hyaluronic acid hydrogel	Designed as a percutaneous intramyocardial injection, shows potential benefit of shear-thinning, self-healing, reduction in myofiber stress post-infarction, sustains natural ventricular geometry and functions	[46]
Extracellular matrix (ECM) hydrogel	Follows intramyocardial delivery, replaces damaged ECM post-infarction, increases vascularization & cell infiltration	[47]
Poly (ester carbonate urethane (PECUU) + epicardial ECM patch	Induces a significant increase in ventricular wall stiffness, alleviates wall thinning, prevents chamber dilation, reduces wall stress	[48]
Cardiopatch hydrogel +human induced pluripotent stem cell-derived cardiomyocytes; (hPSC-CMs)	Mitigates fast action potential conduction to reduce risk of arrhythmias, produces strong contractile forces to support cardiac mechanical pumping, promotes long-term survival *via* vascularization	[49]
Fibrin based tissue patch + human embryonic stem cell (hESC)	Improved cardiac function in conditions of advanced HF following epicardial implantation	[50]
Tissue-engineered vascular grafts (TVEG)	Used for extra-cardiac cavopulmonary shunts in paediatric patients	[51]
Heparin-coated polytetrafluoroethylene (ePTFE) vascular graft (Gore- PROPATEN®)	Designed & marketed as an automated tissue processing instrument used to prepare a stem cell-based biological coating	[52]

(Table 1) cont.....

Types	Features	References
Magnesium-based Bioresorbable Stents	Provide same mechanical force as non-resorbable metallic stents, resorbed within 1 year, no adverse device effects	[53 - 55]

Cardiac Patches

In contrast to regenerative medicine, the clinical use of a cardiac patch is still in its preliminary phase. Cardiac patches, in general, are bilayered scaffolds having a biodegradable poly (ester carbonate urethane) incorporated with an enriched ECM (cardiac) layer. The most commonly investigated cardiac patches are bio-hybrid, sterile, non-immunogenic, isotropic and are designed with an aim to get easily attached to the epicardial surface after light scrapping of the infarcted cardiac regions. The presence of ECM enriched layer promotes endogenous tissues growth (within the patch), host cell recruitment, inflammatory cell regulations, stimulated angiogenesis, formation of new and perfused capillary networks within and underneath the patch treated regions. Thereby, the major advantage of cardiac patches is the hybrid design compared to decellularized cardiac ECM (difficult to affix on infarcted tissues, low mechanical support) and non-ECM containing patches (no significant effects on cell bioactivity and scar formation) [3]. Table **1** highlights various studies on the fabrication of cardiac patches.

Bioresorbable Stents and Scaffolds

Stents are short, narrow, mesh-like metal or plastic tubes that are inserted into the lumen of an anatomical vessel (artery or bile duct) that will open the blocked passage either due to thrombus or embolus. Bioresorbable stents have the potency to overcome the caveats of conventional metallic stents for therapy of cardiac disease (coronary artery lesions). They tend to restore the natural physiology of the vessel wall by maintaining vessel motion and geometry after self-degradation in the lumen (Table **1**). However, they involve a drawback of intraluminal thrombosis, which is basically a by-product of self-degradation even after the completion of the therapeutic process. This may lead to a potential risk of increased thrombogenicity, restenosis and delayed endothelialisation. Therefore, there is an extensive need to evaluate the safety and efficacy of the bioresorbable stents that are planned to be used in clinical practice [3, 11].

Vascular Grafts

Grafting is a process of either joining or untying living tissues surgically. Similarly, vascular grafts are foreign devices that are employed to perform a bypass around an infected artery by a process of diverting bloodstream from one zone to another *via* blood vessels detachment and reconnection. In cardiac conditions such as ischemia atherosclerosis, synthetic grafts often show good potency and efficacy; however, they are associated with potential risks of thrombosis, occlusion and infection. Henceforth, the use of biomaterials-based vascular grafts has garnered global attention owing to their close proximity with cardiac vessels. They are mostly designed to be biomimetic, biocompatible, biodegradable, non-toxic, inert, resilient and resistant to long-term effects of infection, stenosis, calcification and storage. Also, these biomaterials are often embedded with active pharmaceutical ingredients to enhance the biocompatibility and functional properties of vascular grafts (coronary artery bypass and tissue-engineered vascular grafts) [9 - 11].

BIOETHICAL ASPECTS

The use of BMs as a therapeutic modality does not involve just biological or pharmaceutical aspects. The interaction of various fields which may not have a direct relation with the therapy itself but are interwoven in the threads of human life are also considered. Law, philosophy, social relations, technological advances, all equally influence the use of BMs as a therapeutic approach. Such considerations are collectively known as Bioethical aspects, which simply encompass safety, regulatory, and ethical norms for the use of BMs and biomaterial-based regenerative medicines and therapies [56, 57].

Biomaterials: Safety, Regulatory, and Ethical Issues

Safety

The most important parameter for the use of BMs is its safety measure in order to ensure the presence of any unwanted or negative impact on the quality of life of patients. Following are the considerations that have been laid down to scrutinize the role of BMs as safe for human use [56]. (i) First of all, for a material to be considered safe for use, it has to be biocompatible. This means that the material is compatible with the surrounding tissues and body fluids and does not react with them in a way that can harm the body or instigate an immune response from the body. Other than this, the material has to be non-toxic and non-carcinogenic. The material is also to be tested in individuals to see if there are any severe allergic responses that can be fatal. (ii) The effect of temperature can also affect the make-up of many natural polymers. The use of such polymers should be thus restricted to those domains where the temperature does not play an important part. (iii) In cases where animal tissues are being used, the absolute safety of the BMs has to be ensured in terms of bovine or porcine pathogens [57].

Regulatory

The regulatory aspect for the use of BMs is guided by the fact that they should be treated as a therapeutic entity. The selection, procurement, storage, manufacture, testing and marketing should be done with proper regulatory compliance. Standard operating procedures (SOP) and guidelines should be followed at each step. Many natural BMs have shorter shelf life due to their susceptibility towards degradation. The storage and manufacturing procedure of such materials should be decided upon carefully with full consideration of their chemical and physical properties. Apart from these, in the case of natural cells, the working environment should be highly aseptic to avoid any type of contamination (microbial, endotoxins or cross-contamination). The source of each BMs should be carefully authenticated and labeled. Regulations are stricter in the cases where human cells and tissues are used as the issue of bioethics comes into play [58]. Further, the FDA clearing of these products to be used in the market happens in more or less the same way as that of a drug product. The criterion to be fulfilled is different depending upon the use of the product, but the procedure is similar.

Ethical Issues or Bioethics

Bioethics plays an important role in the use of human cells. The concerns regarding the bioethical use of human cells arise from the fact that unlike synthetic or natural but not-human-derived BMs, human cells are a part of the human body which in itself is an identity of an individual. The procurement of human cells is akin to taking away a part of someone's identity [59]. This problem does not arise when one's own cells are used, but in the case of an allograft where someone else's tissues/cells are being used. Proper consent is to be taken before such procurement. In the case of procurement of stem cells from infants or even foetus, consent from the guardian or proper authority is to be taken and which is granted only in selected cases. Other than this, when animal cells or tissues are being used in medicine or as a part of surgical therapy, it is important to mention the source of the BMs in consideration of the religious sentiments of many groups of people [59]. For researches dealing with the use of BMs (natural or synthetic) as well as producers of such BMs associated devices and the medical professionals using these therapies, it is important to keep in mind that the use of BMs in itself is a major advancement in the field of medical science, but by the virtue of the field being so wide, there are many incidences in which the use of BMs transcends from being merely a medical and pharmaceutical approach to a social and cultural undertaking. In such cases, a balance has to be kept between the technological and medical advantages presented by their use and the moral and social dilemmas that come with the use of many materials classified under BM, esp. human cells including stem cells, so that the human race can be served in the best way possible while maintaining the highest level of professionalism [60, 61].

CONCLUSION

Human heart is a structurally diverse and a unique organ that supports the vital functions of a body. However, even slight impairments or disturbances in the normal cardiac rhythm may lead to a variety of clinical conditions that account for 50% of mortality, morbidity and reduced quality of life of affected individuals. The high prevalence of cardiac-related conditions (heart failure, cardiovascular disorders, congenital heart disease, ischemic heart disease, *etc.*) globally has led to advancement in the field of research-oriented cardiac medicine. BMs have recently emerged as a new therapeutic avenue to enhance the process of cardiac repair, replacement and regeneration. BMs are quite unique in nature and the most appropriate BMs are highly flexible, elastic and durable to withstand millions of contraction cycles while eliciting therapeutic actions. Also, they mimic/support the natural functions, assembly & physiology of heart tissues in order to repair and regenerate damaged/impaired heart muscles. Also, the use of BMs has extended to the development of cardiovascular components such as heart valves, blood vessels, scaffolds, gauges, *etc*. BMs can be classified as natural, metallic, polymeric, ceramic and composites depending upon the nature of the source. Owing to their multifaceted nature, the applications of BMs are not limited to cardiac interventions but dwell on a multidisciplinary use in fields as diverse as dentistry, cosmetics, ocular lenses, orthopedics, cancer and diabetes. The most widely exploited and investigated examples of biomaterial-based cardiac regeneration strategies are injectable hydrogels, cardiac patches, vascular grafts, bioresorbable stents and scaffolds. Also, the use of ECM, natural myocardial matrix, as a biomaterial to facilitate the cardiac repair and regeneration has become a prominent area of interest and will continue to dominate in the future as well. With the growing development of BMs, the field of bioethical aspects is also expanding, and it simply encompasses safety, regulatory, and ethical norms for use of BMs and biomaterial-based regenerative medicines and therapies in different fields. In conclusion, owing to their global history of use and leaps made in the areas of research and invention, the progression of BMs will significantly cover new terrains every day with evolving future prospects in the field of cardiac interventions, thereby expanding dependable patient care options with a major goal of improved quality of life.

CONSENT FOR PUBLICATION

Not Applicable.

CONFLICT OF INTEREST

The author confirms that this chapter contents have no conflict of interest.

ACKNOWLEDGEMENT

Declared none.

REFERENCES

[1]   Arnal-Pastor M, Chachques JC, Pradas MM, Vallés-Lluch A. Biomaterials for cardiac tissue engineering 2013.
[http://dx.doi.org/10.5772/56076]

[2]   Ruvinov E, Sapir Y, Cohen S. Cardiac tissue engineering: principles, materials, and applications. Synthesis Lectures on Tissue Engineering 2012; 4: 1-200.
[http://dx.doi.org/10.2200/S00437ED1V01Y201207TIS009]

[3]   Di Franco S, Amarelli C, Montalto A, Loforte A, Musumeci F. Biomaterials and heart recovery: cardiac repair, regeneration and healing in the MCS era: a state of the "heart". J Thorac Dis 2018; 10 (Suppl. 20): S2346-62.
[http://dx.doi.org/10.21037/jtd.2018.01.85] [PMID: 30123575]

[4]   Lam MT, Wu JC. Biomaterial applications in cardiovascular tissue repair and regeneration. Expert Rev Cardiovasc Ther 2012; 10(8): 1039-49.
[http://dx.doi.org/10.1586/erc.12.99] [PMID: 23030293]

[5]   Suuronen EJ, Ruel M. Biomaterials for cardiac regeneration. Cham: Springer International Publishing 2015.
[http://dx.doi.org/10.1007/978-3-319-10972-5]

[6]   Radisic M. Biomaterials for cardiac tissue engineering. Biomed Mater 2015; 10(3)030301
[http://dx.doi.org/10.1088/1748-6041/10/3/030301] [PMID: 26065444]

[7]   Chen QZ, Harding SE, Ali NN, Lyon AR, Boccaccini AR. Biomaterials in cardiac tissue engineering: ten years of research survey. Mater Sci Eng Rep 2008; 59: 1-37.
[http://dx.doi.org/10.1016/j.mser.2007.08.001]

[8]   Park J, Lakes RS. Biomaterials: an introduction. Springer Science & Business Media 2007.

[9]   Parida P, Behera A, Mishra SC. Classification of Biomaterials used in Medicine 2012.
[http://dx.doi.org/10.11591/ijaas.v1i3.882]

[10]   Davis JR. Overview of biomaterials and their use in medical devices. 2003.

[11]   Pignatello R. Biomaterials science and engineering. BoD–Books on Demand 2011.
[http://dx.doi.org/10.5772/1956]

[12]   Hodges AM, Lyster H, McDermott A, *et al.* Late antibody-mediated rejection after heart transplantation following the development of de novo donor-specific human leukocyte antigen antibody. Transplantation 2012; 93(6): 650-6.
[http://dx.doi.org/10.1097/TP.0b013e318244f7b8] [PMID: 22245878]

[13]   Dalmau MJ, González-Santos JM, Blázquez JA, *et al.* Hemodynamic performance of the Medtronic Mosaic and Perimount Magna aortic bioprostheses: five-year results of a prospectively randomized study. Eur J Cardiothorac Surg 2011; 39(6): 844-52.
[http://dx.doi.org/10.1016/j.ejcts.2010.11.015] [PMID: 21193320]

[14]   Byrne GW, McGregor CG. Cardiac xenotransplantation: progress and challenges. Curr Opin Organ

Transplant 2012; 17(2): 148-54.
[http://dx.doi.org/10.1097/MOT.0b013e3283509120] [PMID: 22327911]

[15]   Koh AS, Choi LM, Sim LL, *et al.* Comparing the use of cobalt chromium stents to stainless steel stents in primary percutaneous coronary intervention for acute myocardial infarction: a prospective registry. Acute Card Care 2011; 13(4): 219-22.
[http://dx.doi.org/10.3109/17482941.2011.634011] [PMID: 22142201]

[16]   O'Brien BJ, Stinson JS, Larsen SR, Eppihimer MJ, Carroll WM. A platinum-chromium steel for cardiovascular stents. Biomaterials 2010; 31(14): 3755-61.
[http://dx.doi.org/10.1016/j.biomaterials.2010.01.146] [PMID: 20181394]

[17]   Rigatelli G, Cardaioli P, Giordan M, *et al.* Nickel allergy in interatrial shunt device-based closure patients. Congenit Heart Dis 2007; 2(6): 416-20.
[http://dx.doi.org/10.1111/j.1747-0803.2007.00134.x] [PMID: 18377434]

[18]   van Putte BP, Ozturk S, Siddiqi S, Schepens MA, Heijmen RH, Morshuis WJ. Early and late outcome after aortic root replacement with a mechanical valve prosthesis in a series of 528 patients. Ann Thorac Surg 2012; 93(2): 503-9.
[http://dx.doi.org/10.1016/j.athoracsur.2011.07.089] [PMID: 22200369]

[19]   Akhtar RP, Abid AR, Zafar H, Khan JS. Aniticoagulation in patients following prosthetic heart valve replacement. Ann Thorac Cardiovasc Surg 2009; 15(1): 10-7.
[PMID: 19262444]

[20]   Palmero P, De Barra E, Cambier F, Eds. Advances in ceramic biomaterials: materials, devices and challenges. Woodhead Publishing 2017.

[21]   Höland W, Schweiger M, Watzke R, Peschke A, Kappert H. Ceramics as biomaterials for dental restoration. Expert Rev Med Devices 2008; 5(6): 729-45.
[http://dx.doi.org/10.1586/17434440.5.6.729] [PMID: 19025349]

[22]   Wallace SS. Next-Generation Biomaterials for Bone and Periodontal Regeneration 2019.
[http://dx.doi.org/10.1097/ID.0000000000000939]

[23]   Spadaccio C, Chello M, Trombetta M, Rainer A, Toyoda Y, Genovese JA. Drug releasing systems in cardiovascular tissue engineering. J Cell Mol Med 2009; 13(3): 422-39.
[http://dx.doi.org/10.1111/j.1582-4934.2008.00532.x] [PMID: 19379142]

[24]   Zhang G, Suggs LJ. Matrices and scaffolds for drug delivery in vascular tissue engineering. Adv Drug Deliv Rev 2007; 59(4-5): 360-73.
[http://dx.doi.org/10.1016/j.addr.2007.03.018] [PMID: 17513003]

[25]   Polizzotti BD, Arab S, Kühn B. Intrapericardial delivery of gelfoam enables the targeted delivery of Periostin peptide after myocardial infarction by inducing fibrin clot formation. PLoS One 2012; 7(5)e36788
[http://dx.doi.org/10.1371/journal.pone.0036788] [PMID: 22590609]

[26]   Maya ID, Weatherspoon J, Young CJ, Barker J, Allon M. Increased risk of infection associated with polyurethane dialysis grafts. Semin Dial 2007; 20(6): 616-20.
[http://dx.doi.org/10.1111/j.1525-139X.2007.00372.x] [PMID: 17991214]

[27]   Kütting M, Roggenkamp J, Urban U, Schmitz-Rode T, Steinseifer U. Polyurethane heart valves: past, present and future. Expert Rev Med Devices 2011; 8(2): 227-33.
[http://dx.doi.org/10.1586/erd.10.79] [PMID: 21381912]

[28]   Parrag IC, Zandstra PW, Woodhouse KA. Fiber alignment and coculture with fibroblasts improves the differentiated phenotype of murine embryonic stem cell-derived cardiomyocytes for cardiac tissue engineering. Biotechnol Bioeng 2012; 109(3): 813-22.
[http://dx.doi.org/10.1002/bit.23353] [PMID: 22006660]

[29]   Wang PY, Yu J, Lin JH, Tsai WB. Modulation of alignment, elongation and contraction of cardiomyocytes through a combination of nanotopography and rigidity of substrates. Acta Biomater

2011; 7(9): 3285-93.
[http://dx.doi.org/10.1016/j.actbio.2011.05.021] [PMID: 21664306]

[30]   Pok S, Jacot JG. Biomaterials advances in patches for congenital heart defect repair. J Cardiovasc Transl Res 2011; 4(5): 646-54.
[http://dx.doi.org/10.1007/s12265-011-9289-8] [PMID: 21647794]

[31]   Place ES, George JH, Williams CK, Stevens MM. Synthetic polymer scaffolds for tissue engineering. Chem Soc Rev 2009; 38(4): 1139-51.
[http://dx.doi.org/10.1039/b811392k] [PMID: 19421585]

[32]   Tous E, Weber HM, Lee MH, *et al.* Tunable hydrogel-microsphere composites that modulate local inflammation and collagen bulking. Acta Biomater 2012; 8(9): 3218-27.
[http://dx.doi.org/10.1016/j.actbio.2012.05.027] [PMID: 22659176]

[33]   Chiu LL, Janic K, Radisic M. Engineering of oriented myocardium on three-dimensional micropatterned collagen-chitosan hydrogel. Int J Artif Organs 2012; 35(4): 237-50.
[http://dx.doi.org/10.5301/ijao.5000084] [PMID: 22505198]

[34]   Deng C, Vulesevic B, Ellis C, Korbutt GS, Suuronen EJ. Vascularization of collagen-chitosan scaffolds with circulating progenitor cells as potential site for islet transplantation. J Control Release 2011; 152 (Suppl. 1): e196-8.
[http://dx.doi.org/10.1016/j.jconrel.2011.09.005] [PMID: 22195848]

[35]   Wang Q, McGoron AJ, Pinchuk L, Schoephoerster RT. A novel small animal model for biocompatibility assessment of polymeric materials for use in prosthetic heart valves. J Biomed Mater Res A 2010; 93(2): 442-53.
[PMID: 19569223]

[36]   Cui Z, Yang B, Li RK. Application of biomaterials in cardiac repair and regeneration. Engineering 2016; 2: 141-8.
[http://dx.doi.org/10.1016/J.ENG.2016.01.028]

[37]   Zhao Y, Feric NT, Thavandiran N, Nunes SS, Radisic M. The role of tissue engineering and biomaterials in cardiac regenerative medicine. Can J Cardiol 2014; 30(11): 1307-22.
[http://dx.doi.org/10.1016/j.cjca.2014.08.027] [PMID: 25442432]

[38]   Bar A, Cohen S. Inducing Endogenous Cardiac Regeneration: Can Biomaterials Connect the Dots? Front Bioeng Biotechnol 2020; 8: 126.
[http://dx.doi.org/10.3389/fbioe.2020.00126] [PMID: 32175315]

[39]   Singelyn JM, DeQuach JA, Seif-Naraghi SB, Littlefield RB, Schup-Magoffin PJ, Christman KL. Naturally derived myocardial matrix as an injectable scaffold for cardiac tissue engineering. Biomaterials 2009; 30(29): 5409-16.
[http://dx.doi.org/10.1016/j.biomaterials.2009.06.045] [PMID: 19608268]

[40]   Williams C, Black LD. The role of extracellular matrix in cardiac development 2015.
[http://dx.doi.org/10.1007/978-3-319-10972-5_1]

[41]   Sahito RGA, Sureshkumar P, Sotiriadou I, *et al.* The potential application of biomaterials in cardiac stem cell therapy. Curr Med Chem 2016; 23(6): 589-602.
[http://dx.doi.org/10.2174/0929867323306160303151041] [PMID: 26951086]

[42]   Karperien L, Navaei A, Godau B, Dolatshahi-Pirouz A, Akbari M, Nikkhah M. Nanoengineered biomaterials for cardiac regeneration. Nanoengineered Biomaterials for Regenerative Medicine 2019; pp. 95-124.
[http://dx.doi.org/10.1016/B978-0-12-813355-2.00005-3]

[43]   Reis L, Chiu LL, Feric N, Fu L, Radisic M. Injectable biomaterials for cardiac regeneration and repair. Cardiac Regeneration and Repair 2014; pp. 49-81.
[http://dx.doi.org/10.1533/9780857096715.1.49]

[44]   Ma PX. Scaffolds for tissue fabrication. Mater Today 2004; 7: 30-40.

[http://dx.doi.org/10.1016/S1369-7021(04)00233-0]

[45]   Leor J, Tuvia S, Guetta V, *et al*. Intracoronary injection of *in situ* forming alginate hydrogel reverses left ventricular remodeling after myocardial infarction in Swine. J Am Coll Cardiol 2009; 54(11): 1014-23.
       [http://dx.doi.org/10.1016/j.jacc.2009.06.010] [PMID: 19729119]

[46]   Rodell CB, Lee ME, Wang H, *et al*. Injectable shear-thinning hydrogels for minimally invasive delivery to infarcted myocardium to limit left ventricular remodeling. Circ Cardiovasc Interv 2016; 9(10)e004058
       [http://dx.doi.org/10.1161/CIRCINTERVENTIONS.116.004058] [PMID: 27729419]

[47]   Seif-Naraghi SB, Singelyn JM, Salvatore MA, *et al*. Safety and efficacy of an injectable extracellular matrix hydrogel for treating myocardial infarction. Sci Transl Med 2013; 5(173)173ra25
       [http://dx.doi.org/10.1126/scitranslmed.3005503] [PMID: 23427245]

[48]   D'Amore A, Yoshizumi T, Luketich SK, *et al*. Bi-layered polyurethane - Extracellular matrix cardiac patch improves ischemic ventricular wall remodeling in a rat model. Biomaterials 2016; 107: 1-14.
       [http://dx.doi.org/10.1016/j.biomaterials.2016.07.039] [PMID: 27579776]

[49]   Shadrin IY, Allen BW, Qian Y, *et al*. Cardiopatch platform enables maturation and scale-up of human pluripotent stem cell-derived engineered heart tissues. Nat Commun 2017; 8(1): 1825.
       [http://dx.doi.org/10.1038/s41467-017-01946-x] [PMID: 29184059]

[50]   Menasché P, Vanneaux V, Hagège A, *et al*. Human embryonic stem cell-derived cardiac progenitors for severe heart failure treatment: first clinical case report. Eur Heart J 2015; 36(30): 2011-7.
       [http://dx.doi.org/10.1093/eurheartj/ehv189] [PMID: 25990469]

[51]   Bockeria LA, Svanidze O, Kim A, *et al*. Total cavopulmonary connection with a new bioabsorbable vascular graft: First clinical experience. J Thorac Cardiovasc Surg 2017; 153(6): 1542-50.
       [http://dx.doi.org/10.1016/j.jtcvs.2016.11.071] [PMID: 28314534]

[52]   https://clinicaltrials.gov/ct2/show/

[53]   https://clinicaltrials.gov/ct2/show/

[54]   https://clinicaltrials.gov/ct2/show/

[55]   https://clinicaltrials.gov/ct2/show/

[56]   D'Souza DS, Bhanja A. Bioethical and Biosafety Issues in Biomaterials Used in Oral Rehabilitation

[57]   Saha S. Bioethics and biomaterial research. Trends Biomater Artif Organs 2004; 17: 1-3.

[58]   Sikder P, Bhaduri SB. Regulatory aspects of medical devices and biomaterials 2019.
       [http://dx.doi.org/10.1016/B978-0-12-813477-1.00002-5]

[59]   Nielsen L. Legal and Ethical Aspects of Further Use of Human Tissue. Eur J Health Law 1995; 2: 109-24.
       [http://dx.doi.org/10.1163/157180995X00177]

[60]   Lawrence DR, Rhodes C. Special Issue of Health Care Analysis: Translational Bodies—Ethical Aspects of Uses of Human Biomaterials

[61]   Liras A. Future research and therapeutic applications of human stem cells: general, regulatory, and bioethical aspects. J Transl Med 2010; 8: 131.
       [http://dx.doi.org/10.1186/1479-5876-8-131] [PMID: 21143967]

CHAPTER 10

Biomimetic Materials Design for Cardiac Tissue Regeneration

Manvi Singh[1], Fahima Dilnawaz[2] and Zeenat Iqbal[1,*]

[1] *Department of Pharmaceutics, School of Pharmaceutical Education and Research, Jamia Hamdard, New Delhi-110062*

[2] *Laboratory of Nanomedicine, Institute of Life Sciences, Bhubaneswar- 751023*

Abstract: Globally, heart failure is among the principal cause of death. Heart transplantation is the only way out to replace the diseased or damaged heart. Since this technique has several disadvantages, newer therapeutic approaches are required for cardiac repair. One such approach is cardiac tissue engineering, which helps in designing and developing biomimetic materials that mimic the microenvironment of the myocardium. Approaches for cardiac tissue engineering consists of cell injection, tissue patch implantation, replacement of the valve, and injection of acellular materials. Biomaterials are designed to support stem cell expansion, protection, and differentiation. They also facilitate cell retention, cell survival and provide mechanical support. Advances in nanotechnology have made the biomimetic material design more advanced as it can deliver bioactive factors, manipulate surface topography, control cell behavior, and align cells and tissues properly. Furthermore, electrical conductivity and mechanical stiffness can be modulated as well. Overall, biomimetic materials are the new therapeutic approaches in the field of cardiac regenerative medicine, demonstrating their potential in treating heart disease.

Keywords: Biomimetic, Cardiomyocytes, Electrospinning, Nanofibers, Nanolithography, Scaffolds.

INTRODUCTION

Cardiovascular diseases (CVDs) are a class of diseases affecting the heart and blood vessels, which include two events; heart attack and stroke and are acute in nature and mainly caused by blockage of the blood vessels towards the brain and heart [1]. Heart failure is still the leading cause of death worldwide, killing almost 17.9 million people, which represents 31% of the world's total mortality. In 2015,

* **Corresponding author Zeenat Iqbal:** Nanomedicine Laboratory, Department of Pharmaceutics, School of Pharmaceutical Education and Research, Jamia Hamdard, New Delhi-110062, India; Tel: +91-11-26058689-5662, Fax: 011-26059663; E-mail: zeenatiqbal@jamiahamdard.ac.in

treatment of heart failure alone, amongst the patients suffering from CVD, caused an economic burden of $560 billion [2].

Despite the encouraging use of conventional treatments for heart diseases, the last stage of heart disease is often transplantation or replacement of failed heart. However, this process has several limitations like immune rejection, blood loss, surgical difficulties, and unavailability of the organs for transplantation. These caveats have urged scientists to develop alternative techniques to repair the damaged heart and re-establish its functioning [3]. Cell therapy has also been used as a therapeutic approach to repair the failed heart. In this method, single cells or collection of cells are directly injected into the cardiac muscles, and changes in the heart rate are observed. But this approach limits the treatment of the wounded heart as the rate of cell survival by this method is significantly less, and the transplanted cells are poorly retained. Further, any inappropriate cell source may lead to arrhythmias after cell transplantation [4]. Recently, cardiac tissue engineering has become a great therapeutic approach for cell transplantation in terms of cell injection, cardiac patches, valve replacement, stimulation of endogenous repair mechanism (Fig. **1**).

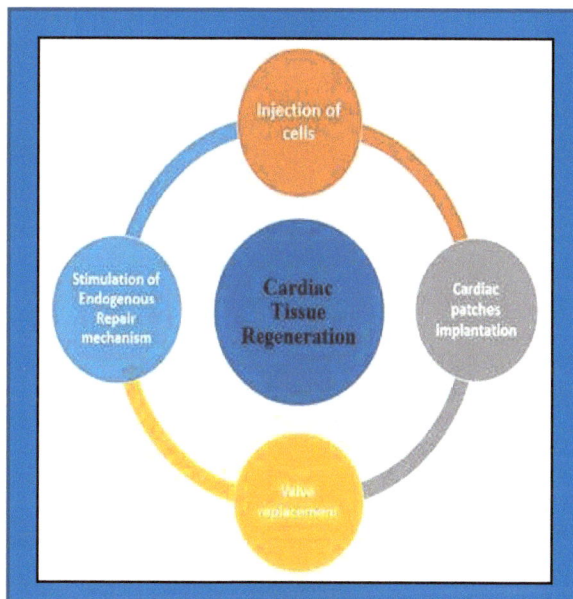

Fig. (1). Various modes of cardiac tissue regeneration.

The development of engineered scaffolds has led to the regeneration of the damaged heart tissue as they provide a microenvironment to the heart cells for expansion and differentiation. They also protect the injected cells into the heart, and their implantation requires surgeries [5]. Tissue engineering has helped in the design and development of biomaterials that mimic the extracellular matrix (ECM) of the heart tissue, and these biomaterials provide features such as molecule adhesion, sequestration, and release of growth factors [6].

Nanotechnology has emerged as an interdisciplinary field involving all the medical doctors, cell biologists, and pharmaceutical scientists for the design and development of biomimetic scaffolds for tissue engineering. Nanotechnology has played a significant role in the development of engineered scaffolds for tissue regeneration. Nano-fabrication approaches have identified goals for nanotechnology, such as functional vascularization, scaffold engineering, and surface-mediated cell assembly [7]. There are distinct advantages of nanotechnology in the preparation of biomimetic materials that may successfully be used for cardiac tissue engineering [7, 8]. Surface manipulation of the individual cell and its structure and function can be regulated by nanoscale topographical features. The chemistry behind the formation of the extracellular matrix can be easily controlled and functionalized. Nanotopography helps in identifying the cellular junction gaps, which in turn helps in cytoskeletal organizations, as a result, the immune response is reduced. Scientists and researchers have taken a step forward in the advancement of nanotechnology as it is capable of manipulating the differentiation of the cell and its behavior by activating the signaling pathways and tracing the differences between the non-functional cells and the cardiac cells. MRI imaging is a key tool in tracking cell migration and development. Liao *et al.* used superparamagnetic iron oxide nanoparticles for *in-vivo* MRI imaging [9]. Different uptake ratios by the embryoid bodies of gold particles are detected through Raman scattering, so they can be used to differentiate between the diverse stages of cardiac differentiation [10]. Furthermore, cardiac biomarkers help stem cell detection by binding to the specific sites, as investigated earlier. NaYF4 nanocrystals were conjugated with the primary antibodies, and cellular junction gaps were detected with the help of near-infrared emission spectra [11]. PEG-PLA-CPLA nanofibers prepared by electrospinning showed two times increased in the expression level of α-myosin biomarker when compared *in-vivo* in an ES-cell derived cardiomyocytes without the nanofibers [12]. PLA nanofibers prepared by rotary extrusion were cultured on neonatal rat ventricular myocytes. These nanofibers showed robust sarcomeric alignment [13]. To form a soft lithography mold, gold-palladium particles were sputtered on a polystyrene sheet in order to coat the mold. PDMS substrates were formed, which directly influenced the orientation of junction proteins like connexin-43 and N-cadherin in cardiac cells derived from stem cells [14].

CLASS OF BIOMATERIALS USED FOR CARDIAC TISSUE REGENERATION

The biomaterials to be used as cardiac repair therapeutics must be biocompatible and biodegradable. They should have reduced local microenvironment hostility and can extend slow and sustained release and facilitate cell engraftment and integration. They must be the putative reservoirs of bioactive molecules. Different natural and synthetic biomaterials used for cardiac regeneration are discussed below.

Natural Biomaterials

Biomaterial for cardiac repair should be either an injectable hydrogel or a patch [15 - 18]. Chitosan is a polysaccharide widely used in food, agriculture, nutrition, material sciences and is also used for environmental protection. Collagen can also be used as a candidate for biomaterial fabrication, as it is a major component of the extracellular matrix (ECM). Alginate is also a polysaccharide obtained from seaweed and used in drug delivery, tissue engineering, and wound healing. Fibrin glue formed from fibrinogen and thrombin helps to create fibrin clots. Some of the natural biomaterials used for cardiac regeneration are listed in Table **1**.

Table 1. Natural biomaterials for cardiac tissue regeneration.

S.No.	Natural Component	Type of Product	Application	References
1.	Collagen	Vitronectin/ collagen scaffold	Cell carrier, induced neovasculogenesis	[15]
		VEGF-collagen patch	Promotion of cell recruitment, increase in ventricular wall thickness, increase in cell proliferation and angiogenesis	[16]
		Collagen patch alone	Increase in infarcted heart contractility due to decreased infarct region fibrosis, improves heart functions, blood vessel formation is increased, decrease in adverse remodeling	[18]
2.	Chitosan	Chitosan gel	Cell scaffold for drug reservoir and carrier, helps in controlled and localized drug delivery	[17]
		Injectable chitosan hydrogel	Helps in stem cell engraftment and survival	[19]
		Chitosan-collagen hydrogel	Endothelial cell apoptosis occurs, structural cell formation takes place	[20]
		Chitosan-hyaluronan/silk fibroin patch	Decrease in LV dilatation, elevated thickness of the heart wall	[21]

(Table 1) cont.....

S.No.	Natural Component	Type of Product	Application	References
3.	Alginate	Injectable alginate-hydrogel	Tissue engineering, increase in scar thickness, drug delivery, decrease in ventricular dilatation, improvement in cardiac functions, wound healing	[22, 23]
		Alginate-chitosan hydrogel	Helps in tissue repair, increased angiogenesis, decrease in cell apoptosis averting LV remodeling	[24]
		alginate-hydrogel in addition to standard medical therapy	Years of benefits in capacity to exercise, decrease in the symptoms, clinical status for patients having advanced HF	[25]
4.	Fibrin glue (fibrinogen and thrombin)	Fibrin glue scaffold	Does not allow infarct wall to be thickened, proper cardiac functioning	[26]

SYNTHETIC BIOMATERIALS

Synthetic biomaterials usually consist of polymers, metals, or both in combination [27 - 30]. They have advantages like good durability and strength, act as a reservoir, enable sustained and controlled drug delivery, support cell integration, but disadvantages such as limited biocompatibility and cell toxicity limit their use. Synthetic materials like Polylactic acid (PLA), poly-glycolide (PLG), and their copolymer PLGA, carbon nanofibers are commonly used for cardiac tissue regeneration. Polyurethane is also used due to its durability and flexibility, and it has the properties to mimic the native cardiac tissue. The self-assembling nature of synthetic peptides helps them to form 3-D hydrogels, which are directly injected into the cardiac tissue for cell differentiation and survival. Some of the synthetic biomaterials used for cardiac regeneration are listed in Table **2**.

Table 2. Synthetic biomaterial for cardiac tissue regeneration.

S.No.	Synthetic Component	Type of Product	Application	Reference
1.	PLGA	Insulin-like growth factor (IGF)-1 bound to PLGA nanoparticles	Increased IGF-1 retention in the tissue, enhanced LV function, decrease in cell apoptosis	[27]
2	Polylactic acid (PLA)	PLA-co-poly(ε-caprolactone)/collagen bio-composite scaffold	Increased cell growth and cell organization	[28]

(Table 2) cont.....

S.No.	Synthetic Component	Type of Product	Application	Reference
3	Carbon nanofibers	Carbon nanotubes with chitosan forming chitosan/carbon scaffold	Increased expression of biomarkers of muscle contraction and electrical coupling	[29]
		Carbon nanofiber/gelatin hydrogel scaffold	Improved results of echocardiography, inhibited ventricular dilation	[30]
4	3D Synthetic peptides hydrogels	Self-assembling peptide puramatrix	Effective cell delivery, improved cell survival.	[31]
		Self-assembling peptide nanofibers as a carrier for platelet-derived growth factor (PDGF)	Cardiac cells are protected from apoptosis, post-MI cardiac function is preserved	[32]
5.	Polyurethane	Polyurethane film	Film pattern is formed, formation of the multilayered contractile tissue construct	[33]

PROPERTIES OF BIOMIMETIC MATERIALS

Biomimetic material can be defined as support or substrate which mimics or matches the microenvironment of the native tissue. These materials may not always mimic the surrounding environment, but their presence may boost growth, engraftment, development, and differentiation of the cardiac cells. Mechanical or structural properties should have the capacity to enhance cell alignment *via* engineered topography, and it should have young's modulus approximately of 0.2-0.5 MPa [34]. The engineered constructs should have applied shear stress and strain as they increase the cardiac cell differentiation [35]. Anisotropic alignment helps electrical contraction and unidirectional propagation. Biomaterials should have proper stiffness and elasticity as defined by ECM composition, and there will be the formation of planned gap junction proteins. Their electrical properties should be conductive so that current propagation takes place through cardiomyocytes, and the myocardium conduction rate should be around 50 cm/s [36]. Their physiological properties should promote cellular adhesion [37], and they should be able to deliver signaling molecules and therapeutics [38]. Furthermore, they should have a capacity for enzymatic degradation [39]; further, from time to time, the synthetic materials used for cardiac regeneration should be replaced. State-of-art methods for biomimetic materials include various methods that are employed in preparing biomimetic materials. Some of them are discussed in this chapter.

Particulate-leaching Technique

This is the most common and easy technique which requires the use of porogens such as sugar, salt, wax, *etc.*, for pore channel production in scaffold fabrication. The material is mixed with the porogen of the desired size, and leaching takes place. After the leaching ends, the matrix is left behind, having pores. These pores can have a size in the range of 300–500 μm and a % porosity of 94-95%. The technique has the advantage of controlling the size and shape of the pores in the scaffold. Thin layers having a thickness of 3mm can be developed with this method [40].

Solvent Casting

It is a casting technology in which evaporation of the solvent takes place, leaving behind a homogeneous film or a scaffold [41]. The solution is made up of a polymer that is soluble in water or a volatile solvent and should be stable in nature and have proper viscosity and solid particles. One of the major limitations of this method is the solvent toxicity which causes denaturation and degradation of the protein. To avoid solvent level toxicity, scaffolds are subjected to a vacuum process and are completely dried, making it a thin efficient film. This method is generally used for preparation of photographic film base, optical films, high temperature resistive films, flexible printed circuits, *etc.*

Gas Foaming

In this method highly porous scaffolds are formed using high-pressure gases [42]. In this technique the polymer used gets saturated and nucleated to form a gas bubble (100–500μm). When high pressure gases are injected into the gas, bubble starts and phase separation occurs. 3-D porous scaffolds can also be formed as no solvent is required in this method.

Sintering/Heat Molding

This technique is carried out in a die set up or mold to form scaffolds [43]. The mixture of polymer/powder and porogen is prepared and added to the mold and is heated above the porogen evaporating/melting temperature or heated above the glass transition temperature of the polymer. Leaching of the porogen takes place, and the scaffold is formed. This process has one major disadvantage as it takes place at higher temperatures, and biologically active moieties cannot be incorporated into it.

Phase Separation

In this method, quenching of the polymers takes place, which results in phase separation of the polymer, termed as polymer poor and polymer-rich phases. The poor polymer phase represents the formation of the porous structure. Porous microstructure formation can be controlled by various properties like polymer concentration, quenching rate and temperature, diffusion of solute particles in the solvent, solvent concentration, solvent type [44]. After the incorporation of bioactive molecules in the scaffold at low temperature, the solvent is either evaporated, extracted, or sublimed.

Rapid Prototyping

The biomimetic materials (scaffolds) fabricated from this technique have excellent accuracy, good mechanical strength, and proteins and cells can be incorporated into it. This technique utilizes computer-assisted manufacturing (CAM) and computer-assisted design (CAD), which comprises selective laser sintering, stereolithography, three-dimensional printing, and plotting [45]. Polymers, ceramics, metals can be used in the preparation of these scaffolds. Disadvantages of this technique are slow fabrication processing, higher temperatures, weak bonding among the powder/polymer particles. These materials have applications in heart valves, cartilages, bone, and adipose tissues.

Freeze Casting

This method involves the development of ice crystals having porous networks. These ice crystals are prepared at a negative temperature by mixing the solute and solvent. After the decrease in the temperature the solute molecules are separated around the ice crystals forming porous network and the solvent is removed by lyophilization [46]. Porous structure of the ice crystals remains intact even after the sublimation process takes place. Benefit of this technique is that the bioactivity of the biological moieties incorporated into the scaffolds are protected and pore size, porosity and morphology can be controlled.

Fiber Mesh

Fiber mesh method involves knitting discrete fibers to form a three-dimensional (3-D) scaffold having different pore size. Advantages of this is enabling the cell attachment and nutrient transport for the cell growth and survival [47].

Electrospinning

Electrospinning helps in the fabrication of nano and micro porous fibers or scaffolds which are helpful in cell binding and other cell activities [47]. These biomimetic materials are capable of replicating the functionalities of the extracellular matrix. This is one of the easiest techniques to prepare scaffolds and more than 90% of the scaffolds are formed by this method. This method involves mixing of polymer in an appropriate solvent and this polymer mixture is filled in a syringe and coated by electrostatic spraying. Various parameters during scaffold fabrication can be controlled in this technique such as molecular weight of the polymer, viscosity, conductivity, surface tension of the polymers, the temperature at which the polymer mixture is prepared, and machine parameters such as flow rate, humidity, temperature, and applied voltage can also be monitored. 3-D scaffolds prepared by this method have properties such as adhesion and adaptability for cell and tissue organization with spatial configuration matching the physiological conditions. These electrospun scaffolds have applications in cell culture for bone and cartilage tissue engineering.

APPLICATIONS OF BIOMIMETIC MATERIALS IN ADVANCING CARDIAC TISSUE REGENERATION WITH EMPHASIS ON NANOTECHNOLOGY

Different approaches have been studied for cardiac tissue regeneration, which includes implantation of cardiac patches, cell injection, replacement of the valve, and various materials are injected for stimulation of endogenous repair mechanism. Biomimetic materials are basically used for differentiation, maturation, and expansion of cardiac cells. These materials also provide structural support to the tissue patches, injected cells, and in developing replacement valves. Cardiac regeneration with the help of nanotechnology can be seen in several examples. Some of them are emphasized here. Davis *et al.*, injected RADA16 self-assembling nanofibers (NF) into the cardiac muscles. These peptides nanofibers were able to assemble themselves in the extracellular microenvironments and promote endothelial cell survival [48]. Controlled drug delivery to the cardiac tissue can be provided by nanofibers containing proteins and peptides [49]. Hsieh *et al.* demonstrated co-injection of peptide nanofiber along with platelet-derived growth factor (PDGF-BB). The combination was able to reduce the death of the cardiac cells. *In-vivo* studies showed that there was a decrease in infarct size in rats having MI and the nanofibers maintained the systolic function in rats [32]. Hashi *et al.* prepared biodegradable electrospun scaffolds incorporated with mesenchymal stem cells. The nanofibers showed remodeling of the matrix and efficient cellular infiltration, just like the native arteries. These nanofibers, when implanted by bypass procedure into the rat carotid arteries, showed excellent long-term patency [49]. Nanocomposite hydrogels prepared from polyvinyl alcohol (PVA) and bacterial cellulose show potential as a biosynthetic heart valve when compared with the native valve [50]. Nanofibrous scaffolds prepared from L-lactic acid and trimethylene carbonate (P(L)LA-co-TMC) increased the proliferation of the cardiac cells and proficiently preserved the morphology of the cell without hindering the expression of a sarcomeric alpha-actinin marker, thus making this synthetic biomaterial potential for cardiac tissue engineering [51]. Stankus *et al.* developed a small diameter duct having integrated cells by electrospinning of a biodegradable elastomer polymer with electrospraying of smooth muscle cells. The vessels developed were flexible and strong, having properties like native arteries, but a disadvantage of thrombogenicity occurs [48]. Topographical evaluation of the valve basement membrane at the nano-scale level was carried out by nanotechnology as it will help in the designing of the scaffolds having desirable properties [51]. Many *in-vivo* studies have demonstrated the advantages of nanoparticles in cardiovascular diseases. Harel-Adar *et al.* prepared phosphatidylserine liposomes injected intravenously to a myocardial infarction mouse model. These liposomes promoted remodeling, angiogenesis prevention of ventricular dilatation [52]. In addition, nanotechnology has also been employed to allow factor and/or cytokine administration in the form of nanoparticles. Anti-P- selectin-conjugated liposomes encompassing VEGF improved the vascular structure and cardiac function in the mice after myocardial infarction [53].

CONCLUSION

The mechanism of regeneration requires extensive research. The collation of bioengineered constructs is quite difficult. The challenging aspects that are faced in preparing these constructs are the biocompatibility, biodegradability, and functionality, as well as the toxicology of the nanomaterials. Therefore, the new therapeutic approach demands the designing and developing biomaterials that precisely target specific sites with different functionalities. Biomimetic materials have advanced surface topography and structures, just like the native cells or tissues. Various methods of nanotechnology like electrospinning, cellular attachment, differentiation, proliferation, nanolithography, and nano-enabled patterning have made it possible to change cell behavior.

CONSENT FOR PUBLICATION

Not Applicable.

CONFLICT OF INTEREST

The author confirms that this chapter contents have no conflict of interest.

ACKNOWLEDGEMENT

FD gratefully acknowledges Dept. of Science and Technology, Govt. of India, for the financial grant [SR/WOS-A/LS-448/2017(G)] in the form of women scientist fellowship (WOS-A).

REFERENCES

[1] https://www.who.int/en/news-room/fact-sheets/detail/cardiovascular-diseases-(cvds)

[2] Dunn DA, Hodge AJ, Lipke EA. Nanobiotechnology, Biomimetic materials design for cardiac tissue regeneration 2014; 6(1): 15-39.

[3] Garbade J, Barten MJ, Bittner HB, Mohr FW. Heart transplantation and left ventricular assist device therapy: two comparable options in end-stage heart failure? Clin Cardiol 2013; 36(7): 378-82.
[http://dx.doi.org/10.1002/clc.22124] [PMID: 23595910]

[4] Dixit P, Katare R. Challenges in identifying the best source of stem cells for cardiac regeneration therapy. Stem Cell Res Ther 2015; 6(1): 26.
[http://dx.doi.org/10.1186/s13287-015-0010-8] [PMID: 25886612]

[5] Thornton AJ, Alsberg E, Albertelli M, Mooney DJ. Shape-defining Scaffolds for Minimally Invasive Tissue Engineering 2004; 77(12): 1798-803.

[6] Buxton DB. Current status of nanotechnology approaches for cardiovascular disease: a personal perspective. Wiley Interdiscip Rev Nanomed Nanobiotechnol 2009; 1(2): 149-55.
[http://dx.doi.org/10.1002/wnan.8] [PMID: 20049786]

[7] Dvir T, Timko BP, Brigham MD, *et al.* Nanowired three-dimensional cardiac patches. Nat Nanotechnol 2011; 6(11): 720-5.
[http://dx.doi.org/10.1038/nnano.2011.160] [PMID: 21946708]

[8] Liao S, Chan C, Ramakrishna S. Stem cells and biomimetic materials strategies for tissue engineering. Mater Sci Eng C 2008; 28(8): 1189-202.
[http://dx.doi.org/10.1016/j.msec.2008.08.015]

[9] Au K-W, Liao S-Y, Lee Y-K, *et al.* Effects of iron oxide nanoparticles on cardiac differentiation of embryonic stem cells. Biochem Biophys Res Commun 2009; 379(4): 898-903.
[http://dx.doi.org/10.1016/j.bbrc.2008.12.160] [PMID: 19135029]

[10] Sathuluri RR, Yoshikawa H, Shimizu E, Saito M, Tamiya E. Gold Nanoparticle-Based Surface-Enhanced Raman Scattering for Noninvasive Molecular Probing of Embryonic Stem Cell Differentiation 2011; 6(8)e22802

[11] Nagarajan S, Zhang Y. Upconversion fluorescent nanoparticles as a potential tool for in-depth imaging. Nanotechnology 2011; 22(39)395101
[http://dx.doi.org/10.1088/0957-4484/22/39/395101] [PMID: 21891842]

[12] Gupta MK, Walthall JM, Venkataraman R, *et al.* Combinatorial polymer electrospun matrices promote physiologically-relevant cardiomyogenic stem cell differentiation. PLoS One 2011; 6(12)e28935
[http://dx.doi.org/10.1371/journal.pone.0028935] [PMID: 22216144]

[13] Badrossamay MR, McIlwee HA, Goss JA, Parker KK. Nanofiber assembly by rotary jet-spinning. Nano Lett 2010; 10(6): 2257-61.
[http://dx.doi.org/10.1021/nl101355x] [PMID: 20491499]

[14] Luna JI, Ciriza J, Garcia-Ojeda ME, *et al.* Multiscale biomimetic topography for the alignment of neonatal and embryonic stem cell-derived heart cells. Tissue Eng Part C Methods 2011; 17(5): 579-88.
[http://dx.doi.org/10.1089/ten.tec.2010.0410] [PMID: 21235325]

[15] Frederick JR, Fitzpatrick JR III, McCormick RC, *et al.* Stromal cell-derived factor-1α activation of tissue-engineered endothelial progenitor cell matrix enhances ventricular function after myocardial infarction by inducing neovasculogenesis. Circulation 2010; 122(11) (Suppl.): S107-17.
[http://dx.doi.org/10.1161/CIRCULATIONAHA.109.930404] [PMID: 20837901]

[16] Miyagi Y, Chiu LLY, Cimini M, Weisel RD, Radisic M, Li R-K. Biodegradable collagen patch with covalently immobilized VEGF for myocardial repair. Biomaterials 2011; 32(5): 1280-90.
[http://dx.doi.org/10.1016/j.biomaterials.2010.10.007] [PMID: 21035179]

[17]   Roughley P, Hoemann C, DesRosiers E, Mwale F, Antoniou J, Alini M. The potential of chitosan-based gels containing intervertebral disc cells for nucleus pulposus supplementation. Biomaterials 2006; 27(3): 388-96.
[http://dx.doi.org/10.1016/j.biomaterials.2005.06.037] [PMID: 16125220]

[18]   Serpooshan V, Zhao M, Metzler SA, *et al.* The effect of bioengineered acellular collagen patch on cardiac remodeling and ventricular function post myocardial infarction. Biomaterials 2013; 34(36): 9048-55.
[http://dx.doi.org/10.1016/j.biomaterials.2013.08.017] [PMID: 23992980]

[19]   Liu Z, Wang H, Wang Y, *et al.* The influence of chitosan hydrogel on stem cell engraftment, survival and homing in the ischemic myocardial microenvironment. Biomaterials 2012; 33(11): 3093-106.
[http://dx.doi.org/10.1016/j.biomaterials.2011.12.044] [PMID: 22265788]

[20]   Miklas JW, Dallabrida SM, Reis LA, Ismail N, Rupnick M, Radisic M. QHREDGS enhances tube formation, metabolism and survival of endothelial cells in collagen-chitosan hydrogels. PLoS One 2013; 8(8)e72956
[http://dx.doi.org/10.1371/journal.pone.0072956] [PMID: 24013716]

[21]   Chi N-H, Yang M-C, Chung T-W, Chou N-K, Wang S-S. Cardiac repair using chitosan-hyaluronan/silk fibroin patches in a rat heart model with myocardial infarction. Carbohydr Polym 2013; 92(1): 591-7.

[22]   Landa N, Miller L, Feinberg MS, *et al.* Effect of injectable alginate implant on cardiac remodeling and function after recent and old infarcts in rat. Circulation 2008; 117(11): 1388-96.
[http://dx.doi.org/10.1161/CIRCULATIONAHA.107.727420] [PMID: 18316487]

[23]   Lee KY, Mooney DJ. Alginate: properties and biomedical applications. Prog Polym Sci 2012; 37(1): 106-26.
[http://dx.doi.org/10.1016/j.progpolymsci.2011.06.003] [PMID: 22125349]

[24]   Deng B SL, Wu Y, Shen Y, *et al.* Delivery of alginate-chitosan hydrogel promotes endogenous repair and preserves cardiac function in rats with myocardial infarction 2015.
[http://dx.doi.org/10.1002/jbm.a.35232]

[25]   Anker SD, Coats AJS, Cristian G, *et al.* A prospective comparison of alginate-hydrogel with standard medical therapy to determine impact on functional capacity and clinical outcomes in patients with advanced heart failure (AUGMENT-HF trial). Eur Heart J 2015; 36(34): 2297-309.
[http://dx.doi.org/10.1093/eurheartj/ehv259] [PMID: 26082085]

[26]   Terashima M, Fujiwara S, Yaginuma G-Y, Takizawa K, Kaneko U, Meguro T. Outcome of percutaneous intrapericardial fibrin-glue injection therapy for left ventricular free wall rupture secondary to acute myocardial infarction. Am J Cardiol 2008; 101(4): 419-21.
[http://dx.doi.org/10.1016/j.amjcard.2007.09.086] [PMID: 18312750]

[27]   Chang M-Y, Yang Y-J, Chang C-H, *et al.* Functionalized nanoparticles provide early cardioprotection after acute myocardial infarction. J Control Release 2013; 170(2): 287-94.
[http://dx.doi.org/10.1016/j.jconrel.2013.04.022] [PMID: 23665256]

[28]   Mukherjee S, Venugopal JR, Ravichandran R, Ramakrishna S, Raghunath M. Evaluation of the biocompatibility of PLACL/collagen nanostructured matrices with cardiomyocytes as a model for the regeneration of infarcted myocardium. Adv Funct Mater 2011; 21(12): 2291-300.
[http://dx.doi.org/10.1002/adfm.201002434]

[29]   Martins AM, Eng G, Caridade SG, Mano JF, Reis RL, Vunjak-Novakovic G. Electrically conductive chitosan/carbon scaffolds for cardiac tissue engineering. Biomacromolecules 2014; 15(2): 635-43.
[http://dx.doi.org/10.1021/bm401679q] [PMID: 24417502]

[30]   Zhou J, Chen J, Sun H, *et al.* Engineering the heart: evaluation of conductive nanomaterials for improving implant integration and cardiac function. Sci Rep 2014; 4(4): 3733.
[PMID: 24429673]

[31]   Tokunaga M, Liu M-L, Nagai T, *et al.* Implantation of cardiac progenitor cells using self-assembling peptide improves cardiac function after myocardial infarction. J Mol Cell Cardiol 2010; 49(6): 972-83.
[http://dx.doi.org/10.1016/j.yjmcc.2010.09.015] [PMID: 20869968]

[31]   Zhou J, Chen J, Sun H, *et al.* Engineering the heart: evaluation of conductive nanomaterials for improving implant integration and cardiac function. Sci Rep 2014; 4(4): 3733.
[PMID: 24429673]

[32]   Hsieh PCH, Davis ME, Gannon J, MacGillivray C, Lee RT. Controlled delivery of PDGF-BB for myocardial protection using injectable self-assembling peptide nanofibers, 116(1) (2006) 237-248. J Clin Invest 2006; 116(1): 237-48.
[http://dx.doi.org/10.1172/JCI25878] [PMID: 16357943]

[33]   McDevitt TC, Woodhouse KA, Hauschka SD, Murry CE, Stayton PS. Spatially organized layers of cardiomyocytes on biodegradable polyurethane films for myocardial repair. J Biomed Mater Res A 2003; 66(3): 586-95.
[http://dx.doi.org/10.1002/jbm.a.10504] [PMID: 12918042]

[34]   Costa KD, Lee EJ, Holmes JW. Creating alignment and anisotropy in engineered heart tissue: role of boundary conditions in a model three-dimensional culture system. Tissue Eng 2003; 9(4): 567-77.
[http://dx.doi.org/10.1089/107632703768247278] [PMID: 13678436]

[35]   Gwak S-J, Bhang SH, Kim IK, *et al.* The effect of cyclic strain on embryonic stem cell-derived cardiomyocytes. Biomaterials 2008; 29(7): 844-56.
[http://dx.doi.org/10.1016/j.biomaterials.2007.10.050] [PMID: 18022225]

[36]   You J-O, Rafat M, Ye GJC, Auguste DT. Nanoengineering the heart: conductive scaffolds enhance connexin 43 expression. Nano Lett 2011; 11(9): 3643-8.
[http://dx.doi.org/10.1021/nl201514a] [PMID: 21800912]

[37]   Tongers J, Webber MJ, Vaughan EE, *et al.* Enhanced potency of cell-based therapy for ischemic tissue repair using an injectable bioactive epitope presenting nanofiber support matrix. J Mol Cell Cardiol 2014; 74: 231-9.
[http://dx.doi.org/10.1016/j.yjmcc.2014.05.017] [PMID: 25009075]

[38]   Sapir Y, Kryukov O, Cohen S. Integration of multiple cell-matrix interactions into alginate scaffolds for promoting cardiac tissue regeneration. Biomaterials 2011; 32(7): 1838-47.
[http://dx.doi.org/10.1016/j.biomaterials.2010.11.008] [PMID: 21112626]

[39]   Benton JA, Fairbanks BD, Anseth KS. Characterization of valvular interstitial cell function in three dimensional matrix metalloproteinase degradable PEG hydrogels. Biomaterials 2009; 30(34): 6593-603.
[http://dx.doi.org/10.1016/j.biomaterials.2009.08.031] [PMID: 19747725]

[40]   Liao C-J, Chen C-F, Chen J-H, Chiang S-F, Lin Y-J, Chang K-Y. Fabrication of porous biodegradable polymer scaffolds using a solvent merging/particulate leaching method. J Biomed Mater Res 2002; 59(4): 676-81.
[http://dx.doi.org/10.1002/jbm.10030] [PMID: 11774329]

[41]   Thadavirul N, Pavasant P, Supaphol P. Development of polycaprolactone porous scaffolds by combining solvent casting, particulate leaching, and polymer leaching techniques for bone tissue engineering. J Biomed Mater Res A 2014; 102(10): 3379-92.
[http://dx.doi.org/10.1002/jbm.a.35010] [PMID: 24132871]

[42]   Nam YS, Yoon JJ, Park TG. A novel fabrication method of macroporous biodegradable polymer scaffolds using gas foaming salt as a porogen additive. J Biomed Mater Res 2000; 53(1): 1-7.
[http://dx.doi.org/10.1002/(SICI)1097-4636(2000)53:1<1::AID-JBM1>3.0.CO;2-R]   [PMID: 10634946]

[43]   Oh S-H, Kang SG, Kim ES, Cho SH, Lee JH. Fabrication and characterization of hydrophilic poly(lactic-co-glycolic acid)/poly(vinyl alcohol) blend cell scaffolds by melt-molding particulate-

leaching method. Biomaterials 2003; 24(22): 4011-21.
[http://dx.doi.org/10.1016/S0142-9612(03)00284-9] [PMID: 12834596]

[44]   Nam YS, Park TG. Porous biodegradable polymeric scaffolds prepared by thermally induced phase separation. J Biomed Mater Res 1999; 47(1): 8-17.
[http://dx.doi.org/10.1002/(SICI)1097-4636(199910)47:1<8::AID-JBM2>3.0.CO;2-L]   [PMID: 10400875]

[45]   Billiet T, Vandenhaute M, Schelfhout J, Van Vlierberghe S, Dubruel P. A review of trends and limitations in hydrogel-rapid prototyping for tissue engineering. Biomaterials 2012; 33(26): 6020-41.
[http://dx.doi.org/10.1016/j.biomaterials.2012.04.050] [PMID: 22681979]

[46]   Deville S, Saiz E, Tomsia AP. Freeze casting of hydroxyapatite scaffolds for bone tissue engineering. Biomaterials 2006; 27(32): 5480-9.
[http://dx.doi.org/10.1016/j.biomaterials.2006.06.028] [PMID: 16857254]

[47]   Zong X, Bien H, Chung C-Y, *et al.* Electrospun fine-textured scaffolds for heart tissue constructs. Biomaterials 2005; 26(26): 5330-8.
[http://dx.doi.org/10.1016/j.biomaterials.2005.01.052] [PMID: 15814131]

[48]   Stankus JJ, Soletti L, Fujimoto K, Hong Y, Vorp DA, Wagner WR. Fabrication of cell microintegrated blood vessel constructs through electrohydrodynamic atomization. Biomaterials 2007; 28(17): 2738-46.
[http://dx.doi.org/10.1016/j.biomaterials.2007.02.012] [PMID: 17337048]

[49]   Hashi CK, Zhu Y, Yang G-Y, *et al.* Antithrombogenic property of bone marrow mesenchymal stem cells in nanofibrous vascular grafts. Proc Natl Acad Sci USA 2007; 104(29): 11915-20.
[http://dx.doi.org/10.1073/pnas.0704581104] [PMID: 17615237]

[50]   Millon LE, Wan WK. The polyvinyl alcohol-bacterial cellulose system as a new nanocomposite for biomedical applications. J Biomed Mater Res B Appl Biomater 2006; 79(2): 245-53.
[http://dx.doi.org/10.1002/jbm.b.30535] [PMID: 16680717]

[51]   Brody S, Anilkumar T, Liliensiek S, Last JA, Murphy CJ, Pandit A. Characterizing nanoscale topography of the aortic heart valve basement membrane for tissue engineering heart valve scaffold design. Tissue Eng 2006; 12(2): 413-21.
[http://dx.doi.org/10.1089/ten.2006.12.413] [PMID: 16548699]

[52]   Harel-Adar T, Ben Mordechai T, Amsalem Y, Feinberg MS, Leor J, Cohen S. Modulation of cardiac macrophages by phosphatidylserine-presenting liposomes improves infarct repair. Proc Natl Acad Sci USA 2011; 108(5): 1827-32.
[http://dx.doi.org/10.1073/pnas.1015623108] [PMID: 21245355]

[53]   Scott RC, Rosano JM, Ivanov Z, *et al.* Targeting VEGF-encapsulated immunoliposomes to MI heart improves vascularity and cardiac function. FASEB J 2009; 23(10): 3361-7.
[http://dx.doi.org/10.1096/fj.08-127373] [PMID: 19535683]

CHAPTER 11

Nanotechnology-Based Direct Cardiac Reprogramming for Cardiac Regeneration

Pooja Jain[1], **Nazia Hassan**[1], **Uzma Farooq**[1] and **Zeenat Iqbal**[1,*]

[1] *Department of Pharmaceutics, School of Pharmaceutical Education and Research (SPER), Jamia Hamdard, New Delhi-110062, India.*

Abstract: Cardiovascular diseases are the main reason for morbidity in developed countries, and congestive heart failure represents the major health burden. Although clinical application of cardiac regeneration is still in its infancy, studies on rodents have proven its feasibility. Also, the technique of direct cardiac reprogramming has unveiled new paths for the success of cardiac regeneration, wherein one cell type can be directly converted into the cardiac myocytes without involving the pluripotent intermediate cell. Firstly designed for the management of cancer, nanotechnology has opened up newer vistas for direct cardiac reprogramming for cardiac regeneration. This chapter discusses cardiac regeneration and the limitations of current approaches to cardiac regeneration in brief. Direct cardiac reprogramming involving both *in-vitro* and *in-vivo* trials has been duly explored to enlighten the readers. An attempt has been made by the contributors to elaborate the various approaches of nanotechnology such as nanomaterials and stem cells in regenerative medicine and their impact on direct cardiac reprogramming. This chapter involves an exhaustive effort of the contributors to enlighten the understanding of a broad readership about the nanotechnology-based direct cardiac reprogramming for cardiac regeneration.

Keywords: Cardiac regeneration, Cardiac reprogramming, Cardiomyocytes, Cardiac fibroblasts, Nanotechnology, Stem cell therapy.

INTRODUCTION

A possible association between nanotechnology and the area of cardiac reprogramming is not limited to textbooks alone. Although still in its infancy, conversion of putative *in-vitro* techniques to *in-vivo* scenarios seems promising and is much required. The limited literature available is suggestive of unravelling certain areas that need to be touched before initiating an effective *in-vivo* evaluation of cardiac reprogramming. These primarily include 1). Identification

---

* **Corresponding author Zeenat Iqbal:** Nanomedicine Laboratory, Department of Pharmaceutics, School of Pharmaceutical Education and Research, Jamia Hamdard, New Delhi-110060, India; Tel: +91-11-26058689-5662, Fax: 011-26059663; E-mail: zeenatiqbal@jamiahamdard.ac.in

Fahima Dilnawaz and Zeenat Iqbal (Eds.)

and characterization of the ideal cardiac resident cell for direct reprogramming. 2). Selective targeting of the injured myocardial tissue with a therapeutically effective dose of reprogramming factor and 3) to achieve the proper *in-vivo* functioning of regenerated cells [1].

The first issue to be resolved is the identification of the ideal cardiac cell for reprogramming. These cells must be in sufficient amount in the heart and easily targetable in the infarcted zone. Furthermore, selective targeting by the nanocarriers, thorough characterization of these cells is the utmost requirement. As after myocardial infarction, infarcted tissue performed a high degree of remodelling process wherein activation of cardiac resident fibroblast takes place, and this attracted the researchers to conduct the study on these cells [2]. Studies have supported these cells as the ideal candidates for direct cardiac reprogramming due to their characteristics, but still, there is a need for further characterization for targeting the nanocarriers [3].

The most suitable combination for reprogramming should be based on the use of chemical entities for which a valid safety profile is available. In order to explore the potential of chemical entities for cardiac reprogramming, a thorough understanding of the chemistry and efficient handling of the customized delivery strategies is needed so that proper administration of compounds with a pre-defined rate can be achieved at the pre-identified target cell. To fulfill the objectives, we need to begin with the identification of material for the engineering of suitable nanocarriers. Biocompatible polymers can be promising materials for the designing of selectively targetable nanocarriers. Moreover, for *in-vivo* efficiency, a more selective strategy of active targeting is required, which can be achieved only after a thorough understanding of the ideal cell candidate. Therefore, the generation of reprogrammed functional cardiomyocytes is the outcome of a combinational strategy involving a cautious selection of the candidate cell and a suitable chemical entity delivered through a suitable nanocarrier [4].

CARDIAC REGENERATION AND LIMITATIONS OF CURRENT APPROACHES FOR CARDIAC REGENERATION

From the last five decades, the center of cardiovascular research lies in the fact that the heart is a terminally differentiated organ, and it cannot replace the functional myocytes after myocardial infarction [5]. In the past 30 years, the focus of research in molecular cardiology revolves around the identification of genes and signaling pathways involved in the hypertrophic reactions of cardiac myocytes during pathologic states [6]. The potential of an adult cell to generate other types of cells beyond its tissue boundary is called developmental plasticity.

Bone marrow cells (BMC) are the most versatile and characterized cell for developmental plasticity in both *in-vitro* and *in-vivo* conditions [7]. Studies were conducted to identify the potential of BMC for tissue regeneration and simultaneously revealed that injury to a tissue encourages the multiplication of alternate stem cells. Based on this, bone marrow cells were injected into the infarcted area of the myocardium or were injected along with cytokines into the systemic circulation. Both the experiments resulted in the repairment of the infarcted tissue and gave rise to functionally active myocardium [8, 9]. Clinical trials have been conducted on human beings for assessing the therapeutic efficacy of BMC in ischemic and non-ischemic cardiomyopathy, and promising results were obtained [10].

By this time, several approaches have been explored to repair the infarcted heart. This includes BMC, fibroblasts, fetal cardiomyocytes, bone marrow-derived immature myocytes, endothelial cells derived from the embryo, skeletal myoblasts, endothelial progenitors, and smooth muscle cells [11]. All of the above-mentioned approaches result in the formation of passive graft by decreasing the negative remodeling, thereby reducing the hardening in the scarred portion of the heart wall. Hence the variable degree of improvement was observed in cardiac performance. However, in a few cases, the dynamically active graft was also observed, which contributed to myocardial contractility [8, 9, 12]. The implanted cells may also exhibit the paracrine response by activating the growth of resident progenitor cells [13, 14].

Recently researchers have identified and characterized the cardiac stem cell in the heart of mice, rats, and dogs [15, 16]. As resident cardiac stem cells involuntarily differentiate into myocytes and vascular structure, these are the preferred cells to be assessed for cardiac repair. C-kit-positive are the self-renewing, multipotent and clonogenic cells having the fundamental characteristics and properties of stem cells [16, 17]. When these c-kit-positive cardiac stem cells with or without local activation factors were injected intramyocardially in Fisher rats, they resulted in significant regeneration of the infarcted heart. In comparison, the IV injection of stem cell antigen 1-positive cell (Sca1) after reperfusion insult resulted in a limited effect on myocardial regeneration [15]. However, it is unclear that the variation in response was due to the route of administration or the distinct progenitor cell. It can be said that myocardial repair requires the regeneration of cardiac myocytes and coronary blood vessels, and this criterion cannot be fulfilled by a cell already programmed for the myocyte lineage. In the absence of blood vessels, myocytes would not survive. Also, the use of cells programmed for exclusively generated coronary blood vessels had not given the significant results of tissue regeneration [18]. For myocardial regeneration, administration of more primitive, multipotent cells is required that can differentiate into variable type of cardiac cell lineages such as myocytes, endothelial cells and vascular smooth muscle cells. Despite the development of well differentiated protocols of stem cell therapy for cardiac regeneration, certain limitations are there to hamper its successful clinical application. The limitations are summarized as below:

Variable Engraftment Rate of Transplanted Cells

Stem cell therapy in treating human disease is majorly associated with low cell survival and low engraftment rate of transplanted cells. The reason behind this is that the grafted cells are not able to withstand the environmental conditions and subsequently triggered the immune response of the ischemic heart. Route of administration of stem cells also has a variable impact on the graft efficiency in the heart. Intramyocardial (IM), intravenous (IV), and intracoronary (IC) are the available routes for direct administration of stem cells into the heart. Although direct intramyocardial administration is the preferred route, it involves a considerable amount of cell leakage from the punctured holes [19]. When an IM implant is conducted through open-chest surgery, it leads to acute inflammation and high-wall shear stress. Contrary to the IM injection, when the cells are injected into the coronary artery, it has shown the minimal possibility of induced ventricular arrhythmias [10, 20]. Although the IV route is considered the non-invasive mean of delivery, it is commonly associated with very poor cell retention as the cells migrate and get trapped into the other organs [21, 22]. In short, whatever be the route of delivery, the engraftment rate of the transplanted cells to the cardiac wall is very poor, *i.e.*, less than 2%. However, several strategies to enhance the engraftment rate are under investigation [23, 24].

Teratoma Formation and Immune Rejection

Following transplantation of human-derived pluripotent stem cells, there is a possibility of teratoma formation and rejection by the immune system. Tumorigenesis is initiated by the presence of residual undifferentiated pluripotent stem cells and poor purification of terminally differentiated stem cells. However, presently no single evidence is there to support the teratoma formation after transplantation, but more in-depth studies involving non-primates 'human models, long-term follow-up after transplantation, and mature cardiomyocytes are required to recheck the safety and efficacy of human-derived pluripotent stem cells [25, 26]. Knowing the fact that most of the studies involving stem cells are conducted on nude animals (immunocompromised), the possibility of stem cell-induced immune reaction in humans cannot be neglected [26, 27]. Although the use of immunosuppressants post-transplantation could enhance the graft acceptance rate, at the same time, the increased risk of infection and malignancies cannot be ignored [28]. It can be concluded that the fact that the heart can accept the stem cells for regenerating myocardial tissue indicates the need for novel approaches for healthy regeneration of the infarcted human heart, which are devoid of any risk. Cardiac stem cells can be grafted and cultured *in-vivo* to the infarcted area of heart for the regeneration of functional myocytes and coronary vessels. A fast and effective regeneration of infarcted myocardium is important for the functioning / survival of both organ and organism. To fulfill this objective cardiac stem cell is a complementary therapeutic approach and represents an exciting scientific endeavour with a long path to travel.

DIRECT CARDIAC REPROGRAMMING

As discussed in the above section, heart regeneration is associated with various difficulties, so in order to regenerate the cardiac cells, direct cardiac reprogramming was introduced. Through this technique, fibroblasts can be directly converted into induced cardiomyocyte-like cells (iCMs) by transducing the cardiac-specific factors [29]. By this, there is no need to first convert the fibroblasts into stem cells, as depicted in Fig. (**1**).

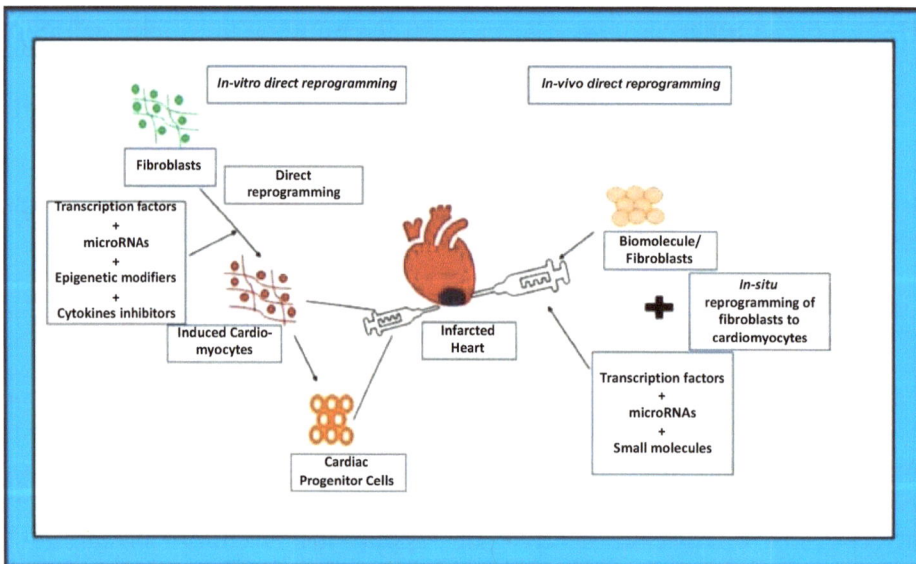

Fig. (1). Schematic diagram representing the *in-vitro* and *in-vivo* approach of direct cardiac reprogramming.

During the procedure of *in-vivo* direct cardiac reprogramming after myocardial infarction, resident cardiac fibroblasts are converted into functional iCMs and improve their activities *in-situ* [30]. Breakthrough in this field comes in 1987, from the study of Davis *et al.* in which he reported the potential of MyoD by directly converting mouse fibroblasts into myoblast, *i.e.*, direct conversion of one type of cell to another [31]. Later to this, the innovative discovery of multiple transcription factors such as Oct4, Sox2, Klf4, and c-Myc by Takahashi *et al.* and Sadahira *et al.* introduced the iPSCs (induced pluripotent stem cell) technology where they demonstrate the conversion of somatic cells into PSCs by multiple transcription factors [32, 33]. This new idea paves the way for the generation of clinically important cells by the introduction of multiple tissue-specific gene cocktail. Zhou *et al.*, for the very first time, exploited the potential of direct reprogramming for converting pancreatic exocrine cells into functional β cells with specifically defined factor combinations [34]. Ieda *et al.* screened 14 key factors and found out that for generating iCMs from CF (Cardiac fibroblasts), factors such as Gata4, Mef2c, and Tbx5 (G,M, and T; GMT)were sufficient. The induced cardiomyocytes showed well-developed sarcomeric structures and multiple cardiac genes like Myh6, Actc1, Actn2 and Nppa [29]. The electrophysiological analysis revealed that iCMs possess similar action potential to that of cardiomyocytes, but after 4-5 weeks, very few cells showed spontaneous contractions. This indicated that only a few iCMs were reprogrammed, and the rest were in an immature state. Thus, despite the breakthrough, cardiac reprogramming efficiency was very low. In another study, Chen *et al.* found out that GMT overexpression through lentiviral transduction was not capable of converting adult cardiac fibroblasts and tail-tip fibroblasts into induced cardiomyocytes, and also the efficiency of reprogramming was very low [35]. Based on the above findings, it can be said that for successful reprogramming, first of all, source cell type and cell conditions are important. And secondly, a proper combination of transduction factors and their high expression levels is required. Thus, for successful reprogramming transcription factors, epigenetic factors and culture conditions need to be optimized [36 - 38].

DIRECT *IN-VIVO* REPROGRAMMING

Although successful attempts have been made by the researchers for conversion of the fibroblasts into iCMs, the potential of direct cardiac reprogramming lies in its *in-vivo* use, where through gene delivery, a large group of fibroblasts can be directly converted into functional cardiomyocytes, as shown in Fig. (**1**). This approach is practicable as *in-vivo* conditions of the heart may help the reprogramming process in a better way as compared to *in-vitro* simulated conditions. Various attempts have been made by the researchers to check the ability of transferred genes of reprogramming factors in infarcted mouse heart to convert the fibroblasts into functional cardiomyocytes *in-situ* [39 - 42].

Qian *et al.* used a retroviral system to express GMT (Gata4, Mef2c, and Tbx5)into mice hearts after coronary ligation and through lineage tracing system showed that even in the *in-vivo* conditions, resident non-myocytes could be reprogrammed into cardiomyocyte-like cells with improved functions. They used fibroblast lineage-tracing mice (Fsp1-Cre and Periostin-Cre) to demonstrate that induced cardiomyocytes are generated from cardiac fibroblasts or nonmyocytes, and α-MHC-MerCreMer mice were used to check whether the newly generated iCMs arose from cell fusion with pre-existing cardiomyocytes. Their study reports that the *in-vivo* reprogramming yield mature induced cardio-myocytes with better efficiency than their *in-vitro* cultures [39].

In a similar study by Song *et al.*, GHMT (GATA4 (G), HAND2 (H), MEF2C (M), MESP1 (Ms), NKX2-5 (N), and TBX5 (T)) retrovirus were injected into the infarcted heart of mice after myocardial infarction, and they reported the reduced fibrosis, improved cardiac activity with the successful *in-situ* conversion of endogenous cardiac fibroblasts into functionally active induced cardiomyocytes [42]. They used Fsp1-Cre and Rosa26-LacZ as noncardiomyocytes alleles and inducible TCF21-iCre mice for fibroblast lineage tracing. They found 2-6% of newly generated induced cardiomyocytes out of all cardiomyocytes in the infarcted area. Electrophysiology, $Ca2+$ transients, and cell contractility procedures proved that new cells have similar functional properties as that of endogenous ventricular cardiomyocytes. The study of Jayawardena *et al.* exploited the potential of miRNA-mediated cardiac reprogramming for cardiac regeneration after myocardial injury. They injected a cocktail of lentiviralmiR (1,133, 208, and 499) into the infarcted heart of the mouse. For lineage tracing of nonmyocytes, Fsp-1 Cre/tandem dimer Tomato (tdTomato) mice were used, and results showed that in the infarcted area, 12% of the cardiomyocytes were newly generated induced cardiomyocytes [43]. All the characteristics features of mature ventricular cardiomyocytes, such as markers, contraction ability, action potential, and presence of sarcomere, were retained by *in-vivo* reprogrammed induced cardio-myocytes. Their study opens the door for the use of miRNA combination instead of transcription factors for cardiac reprogramming. The small size of a single miRNA permits the delivery of multiple transcripts through a single vector, thereby increasing the efficiency and functional homogeneity of newly reprogrammed cells. Also, chemically synthesized miRNA mimics can be more easily administered to cells and are comparatively less toxic to animal models.

DIRECT CARDIAC REPROGRAMMING IN HUMAN FIBROBLASTS

Clinical applications of direct cardiac reprogramming require the successful translation of this technology from mice to humans. Nam *et al.* reported the ineffectiveness of GHMT in activating gene expression of human cardiac fibroblasts, and an additional factor Myocd was required for gene expression in humans [44]. Also, the application of miR-1 and miR-133 (muscle-specific miRNAs) enhances the fibroblasts conversion and excludes the requirement of Mef2c for cardiac induction from adult cardiac, dermal, and neonatal foreskin fibroblasts. Only 10-20% induction efficiency was observed in cTnT-expressing cells from fibroblasts, and only a few cells regenerated from cardiac fibroblasts retained the spontaneous contractility after cell culture of 11 weeks, indicating that mostly induced cardio-myocytes were in the incomplete reprogrammed state [45]. Wada *et al.* reported that GMT alone was not capable of inducing cardiac reprogramming in human fibroblasts. Out of all 11 additional screened factors with GMT, Mesp1 and Myocd upregulated the human cardiac genes with better efficiency than the alone GMT. Although the induced cardiomyocytes did not show the spontaneous beat, they are mature enough to possess the action potential and exhibit synchronous contractility with murine cardiomyocytes when co-cultured [46]. Muraoka *et al.* reported that human cardiac reprogramming could be promoted by the addition of miR -133 with transcription factors such as GMT, Mesp1, and Myocd. With this combination increase in induction of cardiac markers such as α-actinin and cTnT, was noted from 2% to 8% and 23% to 27%, respectively.

Islas *et al.* [47] demonstrated that the combination of Ets2 and Mesp1 reprogrammed the human dermal fibroblasts into cardiac progenitors [48]. These progenitor exhibits cardiac progenitor markers and later divides into cardiomyocyte type cells with cardiac genes, presence of sarcomere with Ca2+ activity in the long term culture environment. All these studies are a forward step towards the clinical applications, but the technique is comparatively less efficient and more tedious than the cardiac reprogramming [49].

NANOTECHNOLOGICAL APPROACHES IN REGENERATIVE MEDICINE

Recent years have witnessed the advancement of nanotechnology and its ramifications in regenerative medicine. As the cell itself is in the nanometer range, hence nanotechnology has the capacity to alter the functioning of organs at a cellular level. For regenerative medicine, the traditional approaches of nanotechnology involve nanoparticles, scaffolds or nanofibers, and nanocom-posites [50]. Upon injection into the ischemic myocardium, PLGA (poly L-lactic-co-glycolic acid) nanoparticle-containing IGF-1 (insulin-like growth factor) has exhibited a reduction in myocardial cell apoptosis by inducing the protein phosphorylation. Also, by reducing the size of PLGA, the complexation of IGF-1 increases and hence resulted in increased Akt phosphorylation activity [51]. It was observed that when scaffolds of higher oxygen-carrying capacity were used to pre-treat the hMSCs *ex-vivo*, it resulted in preferential cardiomyogenic differentiation. Nanofibers, cross-linked with phytic acid, are effective for myocardial regeneration [52]. Also, biomaterial of poly(glycerol sebacate) as matrix polymer and gelatin as outer shell polymer exhibit good cell adhesion, proliferation, and cell-compatibility behaviour [53]. Scaffolds with sub-microscopic and microscopic structures play an important role in myocardial cell adhesion and further growth. Compared to the scaffolds of millimeter and microscopic size range, nano scaffolds provide better bulk and surface advantages [54]. Recently, the role of nanocomposites in cardiac regeneration and tissue engineering is a topic of research for scientists because of their porous nature. The pore walls act as a barrier for cell interaction and hamper the propagation of electrical signals [55]. With the aim to bridge the non-conducting walls, microporous alginate scaffolds containing 3D nanocomposites of gold nanowires have been developed by Dvir *et al.* [56]. These conducting bridges enhance the electrical signal propagation across the cell-seeded scaffolds, thereby promoting the functional activity of the tissue. The potential of nanowires has been explored to increase the expression of connexin-43, which is an electrical coupling protein known to regulate inter-cell communication and promote contractile behaviour [57]. Despite the biodegradable and biocompatible nature, PLGA is also associated with limited cell interaction [58, 59]. Whereas carbon nanofiber composites are conductive in nature, can mimic natural proteins like collagen, and also possess the capacity to transform nonconductive polymers to conductive ones [60, 61]. Due to their nanoscale geometry, they imitate the extracellular matrix of the heart and can enhance the cytocompatibility of pure PLGA [62]. Various studies, as listed in Table 1, have been conducted by the researchers to assess the applicability of nanotechnology for cardiac regeneration, and they observed promising results too.

Table 1. Various nanotechnological approaches and their observed outcomes for cardiac regeneration.

Nanotechnological Approach	Study Method	Study Outcome	References
3D gold nanoparticle based scaffolds	Gold nanoparticles were incorporated inside the macroporous scaffolds to enhance the matrix conductivity and electrical signalling amongst the cardiac cells.	Gold nanoparticles encourage the growth of cardiomyocytes and selectively promote the cardiac sarcomeric actinin expression.	[63]
Carbon nanofibers-based chitosan composite	Development of highly conductive chitosan-based composite with doping of carbon nanofibers.	Increased expression of cardiac-specific genes.Improved cardiac tissue constructions through enhanced signal transmission between cells.	[64]

(Table 1) cont.....

Nanotechnological Approach	Study Method	Study Outcome	References
Hybrid hydrogels containing carbon nanotubes	Dielectrophoresis mediated alignment of carbon nanotubes within methacrylated gelatin hydrogels.	Increased myogenic gene and protein expression due to anisotropic conductivity of hybrid of CNT-methacrylate gelatin hydrogel.	[65]
Gold and laponite nanoparticles loaded myocardial extracellular matrix (ECM)	To investigate the improvement of cardiac function by injectable hydrogel made up of electroactive gold and laponite nanoparticle-loaded myocardial extracellular matrix.	Improved cell compatibility and cardiac specific genes were observed. Study indicates the potential of nanoparticle-loaded extra-cellular matrix for cardiac regeneration post-myocardial infarction.	[66]
Gold nanoparticles dispersed in chitosan hydrogels	Development of electroconductive hydrogels to enhance cardiac cell constructions.	Gold nanoparticles- chitosan hydrogel supported the active metabolism, migration, and proliferation of MSCs. Also, increased expression of cardiac markers was observed.	[67]
GMT loaded gold nanoparticles	Development of cationic gold nanoparticles loaded with GMT genes for *in-vivo* conversion of fibroblasts into cardiomyocytes.	Efficient conversion of fibroblasts into cardiomyocytes was observed upon injection of GMT loaded gold nanoparticles in mice and humans.	[68]

STEM CELLS FOR CARDIAC REGENERATION

In recent years, several approaches, such as stimulation of intrinsic proliferative capacity of resident cardiomyocytes and enhanced differentiation of resident or non-resident cardiac progenitor cells, have been developed to regenerate the functional cardiomyocytes after myocardial infarction. In order to reactivate cardiomyocyte proliferation, researchers have tried to alter the cell cycle barriers by activating the specific cell cycle signalling pathways involved in the differentiation of cardiomyocytes during the development phase, such as neuregulin 1-ErB2/B4 [69]. For heart failure, recombinant human neuregulin 1 (NRG1) is in the clinical trial, and results showed improvement in cardiac activity up to three months; however, the role of cardiomyocyte proliferation in this improved effect is still yet to be explored [70]. One more strategy for restarting the cardiomyocyte cell cycle is the forced expression of cyclins and CDSs (specific cell cycle regulators) [71]. Although this approach was successful in stimulating cardiomyocytes, it led to extensive lethal cardiac damage [72]. Programmed activation of promitogenic genes may give better therapeutic responses than the forced expression of individual cell cycle regulators. This particular objective can be achieved by reorganizing the developmental regulatory pathway, such as the Hippo signalling pathway, which directs cell proliferation and organ size. In a study, Heallen *et al.* showed that the mutational changes in the Hippo pathway enhance the transcriptional ability of YAP1 which interacts with β-catenin on Sox2 and Snai2 genes: thereby stimulated foetal cardiomyocyte proliferation and controls heart size [73]. Another attractive approach to activate the mitogenic program in cardiomyocytes is the microRNA (miRNA). Eulalio *et al.* delivered the hsa-miR-590-3p and hsa-miR-199a-3p *in-vivo* to the neonatal heart post-myocardial infarction. Their observation suggests that the miRNAs promote the proliferation of already differentiated cardiomyocytes in the MI murine model [74]. Researchers have suggested an alternate strategy for cardiac regeneration, which involves the transplantation of cardiomyocytes' progenitor cells derived from different sources or cell types. For this purpose, progenitor pluripotent stem cells, induced pluripotent stem cells, resident cardiac progenitor cells, and non-resident cardiac progenitor cells have been explored as source of transplantable cells [25, 75]. Up till now, randomized clinical trials have been conducted to assess the efficacy of bone marrow derived cells [76, 77]. Although the observed safety profile was good, results showed poor beneficial effects due to poor engraftment rate of transplanted cells and low conversion rate of transplanted progenitor cells to functional cardiomyocytes. Altogether, this allows only marginal improvement of cardiac functions [72]. For the purpose of pluripotent stem cell-based therapies, undifferentiated embryonic stem cells are not good candidates as upon injection into immunocompatible hearts, theyled to development of teratoma, whereas differentiated embryonic stem cell yields stable grafts and hence improved cardiac activity of the rodent [27, 78, 79]. Codelivery of embryonic stem cells-derived cardiomyocytes along with paracrine factors and bioengineered microenvironment promotes the maturation of cells [80]. But due to their immature nature and arrhythmogenesis, reduced efficacy was observed [81]. In the year 2006, a new approach for heart regeneration, *i.e.*, iPSCs, was introduced by Takahashi and Yamanaka, which has opened new windows in cardiac regenerative medicines [32]. Since then, the phenomena of direct reprogramming that involved transforming one type of cell into another, without pluripotent intermediate, came into existence for cardiomyocytes [82]. This phenomenon forced the exploration of transcription factors that could mediate the trans-differentiation of cardio-fibroblast of infarction zones into therapeutically active cardiomyocytes. Both *in-vitro* and *in-vivo* studies have been performed to check the ability of combinations of transcription factors, miRNA and other agents to mediate the trans-differentiation of cardiac fibroblasts into induced cardiomyocytes [83]. Promising results have been observed in *in-vivo* conditions of rodent myocardial infarction models but this strategy needs to be translated into clinical practice for human cardiac tissue regeneration [40, 42].

NANOTECHNOLOGY-BASED DIRECT CARDIAC REPROGRAMMING

Association between nanotechnology and direct cardiac reprogramming is not just a dream anymore. Cell-based therapy, along with the regenerative capacity of undifferentiated cells, *in-vivo* reprogramming of cardiac fibroblasts, and simultaneous release of drugs is a combinational therapy for cardiac reprogramming. Perhaps the use of various smart nanomaterials with nanotechnology may generate advanced therapeutic strategies, thereby will increase the application of nanomedicine in cardiac diseases. In order to explore this potential, Chow *et al.* combined the hiPSC-derived cardiomyocytes with erythropoietin-loaded injectable nanostructured hydrogels and observed reduced cell death and increased remodelling after myocardial infarction. Injectable biomaterials in the form of scaffolds have been used for the delivery of therapeutics such as cells and growth factors to promote endogenous cell repair [84]. Nguyen *et al.* showed that the matrix metalloproteinase (MMP) responsive hydrogel upon enzymatically triggered bio-transformation retained at the infarcted site and can deliver the therapeutics in a sustained manner [85]. Another recently developed approach known as THEREPI can be used for *in-situ* delivery of therapeutically active nanoparticles to increase their efficient retention at the infarcted site. In this strategy, a biocompatible patch can be placed epicardially on the border area of the infarcted heart so that drugs, macromolecules, and cells can be delivered in a sustained manner for cardiac therapy [86]. In the case of ischemic cardiomyopathies, the enhanced permeability and retention (EPR) effect can be potentially used to improve therapeutic delivery. During the initial stages of post-myocardial infarction, blood vessels resemble tumor development, such as capillary sprouting, excess vessel branching, endothelial cell proliferation, distorted and enlarged vessels giving rise to leaky vasculature [87, 88]. By utilizing this morphology, nanoparticles can be specifically targeted at the diseased area, and this has been proven to be reproducible in myocardial infarction [89]. Although poor results are observed with the mature fibrotic scar, soon after infarction [90], EPR phenomena will serve as a promising approach that can be translated to clinics in the future for successful myocardial infarction treatment. Apart from the availability of innovative materials and approaches for improved therapeutic delivery, the exploration of a new strategy for cardiac homeostasis is the demand for reversing cardiac dysfunction. Aiming to this, modifications of cardiac metabolism, cardiac-specific gene expressions, and miRNA-mediated therapy represents the new breakthrough for cardiovascular disease treatment [91]. For the development of new therapies and in order to access the potential toxicity of nanomaterials, disease modelling, and *in-vitro* to *in-vivo* translation of pharmacological activities, practical physiological-like tissue models are of utmost consideration. Conventional pre-clinical screenings involve single-layer cells on two-dimensional rigid surfaces or study on animal models, which may not always correctly mimics human physiology. Instead of these conventional strategies, organ-on-a-chip technology is a new promising approach, where three-dimensional cell biology is taken as a base and combined with the recent microfluidic advances to provide human organ-like physiology and tissue level responses [49, 50].

CONCLUSION

Although still in its initial stage, direct cardiac reprogramming has undergone several developments due to nanotechnology-based approaches such as nanomaterials and stem cells. From a clinical perspective, direct cardiac reprogramming holds remarkable potential for treating cardiovascular diseases with patient-specific drug screening, cardiac disease modeling, and regeneration of the infarcted heart. Despite benefits, further studies on human candidates involving nanotechnological approaches for direct cardiac reprogramming are still needed to validate its therapeutic efficacy. But with the advancement of nanotechnology, it can be assumed that in the near future, the efficacy and success rate of cardiac regeneration will increase at a very fast pace.

CONSENT FOR PUBLICATION

Not Applicable.

CONFLICT OF INTEREST

The author confirms that this chapter contents have no conflict of interest.

ACKNOWLEDGEMENT

"Pooja Jain is thankful to Jamia Hamdard for providing Jamia Hamdard-Silver Jubilee research fellowship-2017, AS/Fellow/JH-5/2018".

REFERENCES

[1]   Passaro F, Testa G, Ambrosone L, *et al.* Nanotechnology-based cardiac targeting and direct cardiac reprogramming: the betrothed 2017.
[http://dx.doi.org/10.1155/2017/4940397]

[2]   Tallquist MD, Molkentin JD. Redefining the identity of cardiac fibroblasts. Nat Rev Cardiol 2017; 14(8): 484-91.
[http://dx.doi.org/10.1038/nrcardio.2017.57] [PMID: 28436487]

[3]   Ma Y, Iyer RP, Jung M, Czubryt MP, Lindsey ML. Cardiac Fibroblast Activation Post-Myocardial Infarction: Current Knowledge Gaps. Trends Pharmacol Sci 2017; 38(5): 448-58.
[http://dx.doi.org/10.1016/j.tips.2017.03.001] [PMID: 28365093]

[4]   Sadahiro T, Yamanaka S, Ieda M. Direct cardiac reprogramming: progress and challenges in basic biology and clinical applications. Circ Res 2015; 116(8): 1378-91.
[http://dx.doi.org/10.1161/CIRCRESAHA.116.305374] [PMID: 25858064]

[5]   MacLellan WR, Schneider MD. Genetic dissection of cardiac growth control pathways. Annu Rev

Physiol 2000; 62: 289-319.
[http://dx.doi.org/10.1146/annurev.physiol.62.1.289] [PMID: 10845093]

[6]   Chien KR, Karsenty G. Longevity and lineages: toward the integrative biology of degenerative diseases in heart, muscle, and bone. Cell 2005; 120(4): 533-44.
[http://dx.doi.org/10.1016/j.cell.2005.02.006] [PMID: 15734685]

[7]   Anversa P, Leri A, Kajstura J. Cardiac regeneration. J Am Coll Cardiol 2006; 47(9): 1769-76.
[http://dx.doi.org/10.1016/j.jacc.2006.02.003] [PMID: 16682300]

[8]   Orlic D, Kajstura J, Chimenti S, *et al.* Bone marrow cells regenerate infarcted myocardium. Nature 2001; 410(6829): 701-5.
[http://dx.doi.org/10.1038/35070587] [PMID: 11287958]

[9]   Orlic D, Kajstura J, Chimenti S, *et al.* Mobilized bone marrow cells repair the infarcted heart, improving function and survival. Proc Natl Acad Sci USA 2001; 98(18): 10344-9.
[http://dx.doi.org/10.1073/pnas.181177898] [PMID: 11504914]

[10]   Wollert KC, Drexler H. Clinical applications of stem cells for the heart. Circ Res 2005; 96(2): 151-63.
[http://dx.doi.org/10.1161/01.RES.0000155333.69009.63] [PMID: 15692093]

[11]   Urbanek K, Torella D, Sheikh F, *et al.* Myocardial regeneration by activation of multipotent cardiac stem cells in ischemic heart failure. Proc Natl Acad Sci USA 2005; 102(24): 8692-7.
[http://dx.doi.org/10.1073/pnas.0500169102] [PMID: 15932947]

[12]   Kajstura J, Rota M, Whang B, *et al.* Bone marrow cells differentiate in cardiac cell lineages after infarction independently of cell fusion. Circ Res 2005; 96(1): 127-37.
[http://dx.doi.org/10.1161/01.RES.0000151843.79801.60] [PMID: 15569828]

[13]   Yoon Y-S, Wecker A, Heyd L, *et al.* Clonally expanded novel multipotent stem cells from human bone marrow regenerate myocardium after myocardial infarction. J Clin Invest 2005; 115(2): 326-38.
[http://dx.doi.org/10.1172/JCI200522326] [PMID: 15690083]

[14]   Behfar A, Zingman LV, Hodgson DM, *et al.* Stem cell differentiation requires a paracrine pathway in the heart. FASEB J 2002; 16(12): 1558-66.
[http://dx.doi.org/10.1096/fj.02-0072com] [PMID: 12374778]

[15]   Oh H, Bradfute SB, Gallardo TD, *et al.* Cardiac progenitor cells from adult myocardium: homing, differentiation, and fusion after infarction. Proc Natl Acad Sci USA 2003; 100(21): 12313-8.
[http://dx.doi.org/10.1073/pnas.2132126100] [PMID: 14530411]

[16]   Linke A, Müller P, Nurzynska D, *et al.* Stem cells in the dog heart are self-renewing, clonogenic, and multipotent and regenerate infarcted myocardium, improving cardiac function. Proc Natl Acad Sci USA 2005; 102(25): 8966-71.
[http://dx.doi.org/10.1073/pnas.0502678102] [PMID: 15951423]

[17]   Beltrami AP, Barlucchi L, Torella D, *et al.* Adult cardiac stem cells are multipotent and support myocardial regeneration. Cell 2003; 114(6): 763-76.
[http://dx.doi.org/10.1016/S0092-8674(03)00687-1] [PMID: 14505575]

[18]   Chien KR. Stem cells: lost in translation. Nature 2004; 428(6983): 607-8.
[http://dx.doi.org/10.1038/nature02500] [PMID: 15034595]

[19]   Liew LC, Ho BX, Soh BS. Mending a broken heart: current strategies and limitations of cell-based therapy. Stem Cell Res Ther 2020; 11(1): 138.
[http://dx.doi.org/10.1186/s13287-020-01648-0] [PMID: 32216837]

[20]   Fukushima S, Varela-Carver A, Coppen SR, *et al.* Direct intramyocardial but not intracoronary injection of bone marrow cells induces ventricular arrhythmias in a rat chronic ischemic heart failure model. Circulation 2007; 115(17): 2254-61.
[http://dx.doi.org/10.1161/CIRCULATIONAHA.106.662577] [PMID: 17438152]

[21]   Brenner W, Aicher A, Eckey T, *et al.* 111In-labeled CD34+ hematopoietic progenitor cells in a rat

myocardial infarction model. J Nucl Med 2004; 45(3): 512-8.
[PMID: 15001696]

[22]   Forest VF, Tirouvanziam AM, Perigaud C, *et al.* Heymann M-F M, Crochet DP, Lemarchand P. Cell distribution after intracoronary bone marrow stem cell delivery in damaged and undamaged myocardium: implications for clinical trials. Stem Cell Res Ther 2010; 1(4): 1-11.

[23]   Zeng L, Hu Q, Wang X, Mansoor A, Lee J, Feygin J. 2007; 115(14): 1866-75.

[24]   Hong KU, Li Q-H, Guo Y, *et al.* A highly sensitive and accurate method to quantify absolute numbers of c-kit+ cardiac stem cells following transplantation in mice. Basic Res Cardiol 2013; 108(3): 346.
[http://dx.doi.org/10.1007/s00395-013-0346-0] [PMID: 23549981]

[25]   Chong JJH, Yang X, Don CW, *et al.* Human embryonic-stem-cell-derived cardiomyocytes regenerate non-human primate hearts. Nature 2014; 510(7504): 273-7.
[http://dx.doi.org/10.1038/nature13233] [PMID: 24776797]

[26]   Shiba Y, Fernandes S, Zhu W-Z, *et al.* Human ES-cell-derived cardiomyocytes electrically couple and suppress arrhythmias in injured hearts. Nature 2012; 489(7415): 322-5.
[http://dx.doi.org/10.1038/nature11317] [PMID: 22864415]

[27]   Laflamme MA, Chen KY, Naumova AV, *et al.* Cardiomyocytes derived from human embryonic stem cells in pro-survival factors enhance function of infarcted rat hearts. Nat Biotechnol 2007; 25(9): 1015-24.
[http://dx.doi.org/10.1038/nbt1327] [PMID: 17721512]

[28]   Chinen J, Buckley RH. Transplantation immunology: solid organ and bone marrow. J Allergy Clin Immunol 2010; 125(2) (Suppl. 2): S324-35.
[http://dx.doi.org/10.1016/j.jaci.2009.11.014] [PMID: 20176267]

[29]   Ieda M, Fu J-D, Delgado-Olguin P, *et al.* Direct reprogramming of fibroblasts into functional cardiomyocytes by defined factors. Cell 2010; 142(3): 375-86.
[http://dx.doi.org/10.1016/j.cell.2010.07.002] [PMID: 20691899]

[30]   Tani H, Sadahiro T, Ieda M. Direct cardiac reprogramming: a novel approach for heart regeneration 2018.
[http://dx.doi.org/10.3390/ijms19092629]

[31]   Davis RL, Weintraub H, Lassar AB. Expression of a single transfected cDNA converts fibroblasts to myoblasts. Cell 1987; 51(6): 987-1000.
[http://dx.doi.org/10.1016/0092-8674(87)90585-X] [PMID: 3690668]

[32]   Takahashi K, Yamanaka S. Induction of pluripotent stem cells from mouse embryonic and adult fibroblast cultures by defined factors. Cell 2006; 126(4): 663-76.
[http://dx.doi.org/10.1016/j.cell.2006.07.024] [PMID: 16904174]

[33]   Sadahiro T, Yamanaka S, Ieda M. Direct cardiac reprogramming: progress and challenges in basic biology and clinical applications. Circ Res 2015; 116(8): 1378-91.
[http://dx.doi.org/10.1161/CIRCRESAHA.116.305374] [PMID: 25858064]

[34]   Zhou Q, Brown J, Kanarek A, Rajagopal J, Melton DA. *In vivo* reprogramming of adult pancreatic exocrine cells to β-cells. Nature 2008; 455(7213): 627-32.
[http://dx.doi.org/10.1038/nature07314] [PMID: 18754011]

[35]   Chen JX, Krane M, Deutsch M-A, *et al.* Inefficient reprogramming of fibroblasts into cardiomyocytes using Gata4, Mef2c, and Tbx5. Circ Res 2012; 111(1): 50-5.
[http://dx.doi.org/10.1161/CIRCRESAHA.112.270264] [PMID: 22581928]

[36]   Polo JM, Anderssen E, Walsh RM, *et al.* A molecular roadmap of reprogramming somatic cells into iPS cells. Cell 2012; 151(7): 1617-32.
[http://dx.doi.org/10.1016/j.cell.2012.11.039] [PMID: 23260147]

[37]   Carey BW, Markoulaki S, Hanna JH, *et al.* Reprogramming factor stoichiometry influences the

epigenetic state and biological properties of induced pluripotent stem cells. Cell Stem Cell 2011; 9(6): 588-98.
[http://dx.doi.org/10.1016/j.stem.2011.11.003] [PMID: 22136932]

[38]   Takahashi K, Okita K, Nakagawa M, Yamanaka S. Induction of pluripotent stem cells from fibroblast cultures. Nat Protoc 2007; 2(12): 3081-9.
[http://dx.doi.org/10.1038/nprot.2007.418] [PMID: 18079707]

[39]   Qian L, Huang Y, Spencer CI, *et al. In vivo* reprogramming of murine cardiac fibroblasts into induced cardiomyocytes. Nature 2012; 485(7400): 593-8.
[http://dx.doi.org/10.1038/nature11044] [PMID: 22522929]

[40]   Inagawa K, Miyamoto K, Yamakawa H, *et al.* Induction of cardiomyocyte-like cells in infarct hearts by gene transfer of Gata4, Mef2c, and Tbx5. Circ Res 2012; 111(9): 1147-56.
[http://dx.doi.org/10.1161/CIRCRESAHA.112.271148] [PMID: 22931955]

[41]   Mathison M, Gersch RP, Nasser A, *et al. In vivo* cardiac cellular reprogramming efficacy is enhanced by angiogenic preconditioning of the infarcted myocardium with vascular endothelial growth factor. J Am Heart Assoc 2012; 1(6)e005652
[http://dx.doi.org/10.1161/JAHA.112.005652] [PMID: 23316332]

[42]   Song K, Nam Y-J, Luo X, *et al.* Heart repair by reprogramming non-myocytes with cardiac transcription factors. Nature 2012; 485(7400): 599-604.
[http://dx.doi.org/10.1038/nature11139] [PMID: 22660318]

[43]   Jayawardena TM, Finch EA, Zhang L, *et al.* MicroRNA induced cardiac reprogramming *in vivo*: evidence for mature cardiac myocytes and improved cardiac function. Circ Res 2015; 116(3): 418-24.
[http://dx.doi.org/10.1161/CIRCRESAHA.116.304510] [PMID: 25351576]

[44]   Nam Y-J, Song K, Luo X, *et al.* Reprogramming of human fibroblasts toward a cardiac fate. Proc Natl Acad Sci USA 2013; 110(14): 5588-93.
[http://dx.doi.org/10.1073/pnas.1301019110] [PMID: 23487791]

[45]   Liu N, Bezprozvannaya S, Williams AH, *et al.* microRNA-133a regulates cardiomyocyte proliferation and suppresses smooth muscle gene expression in the heart. Genes Dev 2008; 22(23): 3242-54.
[http://dx.doi.org/10.1101/gad.1738708] [PMID: 19015276]

[46]   Wada R, Muraoka N, Inagawa K, *et al.* Induction of human cardiomyocyte-like cells from fibroblasts by defined factors. Proc Natl Acad Sci USA 2013; 110(31): 12667-72.
[http://dx.doi.org/10.1073/pnas.1304053110] [PMID: 23861494]

[47]   Muraoka N, Yamakawa H, Miyamoto K, *et al.* MiR-133 promotes cardiac reprogramming by directly repressing Snail and silencing fibroblast signatures. EMBO J 2014; 33(14): 1565-81.
[http://dx.doi.org/10.15252/embj.201387605] [PMID: 24920580]

[48]   Islas JF, Liu Y, Weng K-C, *et al.* Transcription factors ETS2 and MESP1 transdifferentiate human dermal fibroblasts into cardiac progenitors. Proc Natl Acad Sci USA 2012; 109(32): 13016-21.
[http://dx.doi.org/10.1073/pnas.1120299109] [PMID: 22826236]

[49]   Nam Y-J, Song K, Olson EN. Heart repair by cardiac reprogramming. Nat Med 2013; 19(4): 413-5.
[http://dx.doi.org/10.1038/nm.3147] [PMID: 23558630]

[50]   Chaudhury K, Kumar V, Kandasamy J, RoyChoudhury S. Regenerative nanomedicine: current perspectives and future directions. Int J Nanomedicine 2014; 9: 4153-67.
[http://dx.doi.org/10.2147/IJN.S45332] [PMID: 25214780]

[51]   Chang M-Y, Yang Y-J, Chang C-H, *et al.* Functionalized nanoparticles provide early cardioprotection after acute myocardial infarction. J Control Release 2013; 170(2): 287-94.
[http://dx.doi.org/10.1016/j.jconrel.2013.04.022] [PMID: 23665256]

[52]   Ravichandran R, Seitz V, Reddy Venugopal J, *et al.* Mimicking native extracellular matrix with phytic acid-crosslinked protein nanofibers for cardiac tissue engineering. Macromol Biosci 2013; 13(3): 366-75.

[http://dx.doi.org/10.1002/mabi.201200391] [PMID: 23335565]

[53]   Ravichandran R, Venugopal JR, Sundarrajan S, Mukherjee S, Ramakrishna S. Poly(Glycerol sebacate)/gelatin core/shell fibrous structure for regeneration of myocardial infarction. Tissue Eng Part A 2011; 17(9-10): 1363-73.
[http://dx.doi.org/10.1089/ten.tea.2010.0441] [PMID: 21247338]

[54]   Webster TJ, Schadler LS, Siegel RW, Bizios R. Mechanisms of enhanced osteoblast adhesion on nanophase alumina involve vitronectin. Tissue Eng 2001; 7(3): 291-301.
[http://dx.doi.org/10.1089/107632701152044152] [PMID: 11429149]

[55]   Bursac N, Loo Y, Leong K, Tung L. Novel anisotropic engineered cardiac tissues: studies of electrical propagation. Biochem Biophys Res Commun 2007; 361(4): 847-53.
[http://dx.doi.org/10.1016/j.bbrc.2007.07.138] [PMID: 17689494]

[56]   Dvir T, Timko BP, Brigham MD, *et al.* Nanowired three-dimensional cardiac patches. Nat Nanotechnol 2011; 6(11): 720-5.
[http://dx.doi.org/10.1038/nnano.2011.160] [PMID: 21946708]

[57]   Ando M, Katare RG, Kakinuma Y, *et al.* Efferent vagal nerve stimulation protects heart against ischemia-induced arrhythmias by preserving connexin43 protein. Circulation 2005; 112(2): 164-70.
[http://dx.doi.org/10.1161/CIRCULATIONAHA.104.525493] [PMID: 15998674]

[58]   Joachim Loo SC, Jason Tan WL, Khoa SM, Chia NK, Venkatraman S, Boey F. Hydrolytic degradation characteristics of irradiated multi-layered PLGA films. Int J Pharm 2008; 360(1-2): 228-30.
[http://dx.doi.org/10.1016/j.ijpharm.2008.04.017] [PMID: 18514448]

[59]   Koh LB, Rodriguez I, Zhou J. Platelet adhesion studies on nanostructured poly(lactic-co-glycol-c-acid)-carbon nanotube composite. J Biomed Mater Res A 2008; 86(2): 394-401.
[http://dx.doi.org/10.1002/jbm.a.31605] [PMID: 17969028]

[60]   Beachley V, Wen X. Polymer nanofibrous structures: Fabrication, biofunctionalization, and cell interactions. Prog Polym Sci 2010; 35(7): 868-92.
[http://dx.doi.org/10.1016/j.progpolymsci.2010.03.003] [PMID: 20582161]

[61]   Liang D, Hsiao BS, Chu B. Functional electrospun nanofibrous scaffolds for biomedical applications. Adv Drug Deliv Rev 2007; 59(14): 1392-412.
[http://dx.doi.org/10.1016/j.addr.2007.04.021] [PMID: 17884240]

[62]   Tran PA, Zhang L, Webster TJ. Carbon nanofibers and carbon nanotubes in regenerative medicine. Adv Drug Deliv Rev 2009; 61(12): 1097-114.
[http://dx.doi.org/10.1016/j.addr.2009.07.010] [PMID: 19647768]

[63]   Shevach M, Maoz BM, Feiner R, Shapira A, Dvir T. Nanoengineering gold particle composite fibers for cardiac tissue engineering. J Mater Chem B Mater Biol Med 2013; 1(39): 5210-7.
[http://dx.doi.org/10.1039/c3tb20584c] [PMID: 32263327]

[64]   Martins AM, Eng G, Caridade SG, Mano JF, Reis RL, Vunjak-Novakovic G. Electrically conductive chitosan/carbon scaffolds for cardiac tissue engineering. Biomacromolecules 2014; 15(2): 635-43.
[http://dx.doi.org/10.1021/bm401679q] [PMID: 24417502]

[65]   Ahadian S, Ramón-Azcón J, Estili M, *et al.* Hybrid hydrogels containing vertically aligned carbon nanotubes with anisotropic electrical conductivity for muscle myofiber fabrication. Sci Rep 2014; 4: 4271.
[http://dx.doi.org/10.1038/srep04271] [PMID: 24642903]

[66]   Zhang Y, Fan W, Wang K, Wei H, Zhang R, Wu Y. Novel preparation of Au nanoparticles loaded Laponite nanoparticles/ECM injectable hydrogel on cardiac differentiation of resident cardiac stem cells to cardiomyocytes. J Photochem Photobiol B 2019; 192: 49-54.
[http://dx.doi.org/10.1016/j.jphotobiol.2018.12.022] [PMID: 30682654]

[67]   Baei P, Jalili-Firoozinezhad S, Rajabi-Zeleti S, Tafazzoli-Shadpour M, Baharvand H, Aghdami N.

Electrically conductive gold nanoparticle-chitosan thermosensitive hydrogels for cardiac tissue engineering. Mater Sci Eng C 2016; 63: 131-41.
[http://dx.doi.org/10.1016/j.msec.2016.02.056] [PMID: 27040204]

[68]   Chang Y, Lee E, Kim J, Kwon Y-W, Kwon Y, Kim J. Efficient *in vivo* direct conversion of fibroblasts into cardiomyocytes using a nanoparticle-based gene carrier. Biomaterials 2019; 192: 500-9.
[http://dx.doi.org/10.1016/j.biomaterials.2018.11.034] [PMID: 30513475]

[69]   Bersell K, Arab S, Haring B, Kühn B. Neuregulin1/ErbB4 signaling induces cardiomyocyte proliferation and repair of heart injury. Cell 2009; 138(2): 257-70.
[http://dx.doi.org/10.1016/j.cell.2009.04.060] [PMID: 19632177]

[70]   Jabbour A, Hayward CS, Keogh AM, *et al.* Parenteral administration of recombinant human neuregulin-1 to patients with stable chronic heart failure produces favourable acute and chronic haemodynamic responses. Eur J Heart Fail 2011; 13(1): 83-92.
[http://dx.doi.org/10.1093/eurjhf/hfq152] [PMID: 20810473]

[71]   Hassink RJ, Pasumarthi KB, Nakajima H, *et al.* Cardiomyocyte cell cycle activation improves cardiac function after myocardial infarction. Cardiovasc Res 2008; 78(1): 18-25.
[http://dx.doi.org/10.1093/cvr/cvm101] [PMID: 18079102]

[72]   Lin Z, Pu WT. Strategies for cardiac regeneration and repair 2014.
[http://dx.doi.org/10.1126/scitranslmed.3006681]

[73]   Heallen T, Zhang M, Wang J, *et al.* Hippo pathway inhibits Wnt signaling to restrain cardiomyocyte proliferation and heart size. Science 2011; 332(6028): 458-61.
[http://dx.doi.org/10.1126/science.1199010] [PMID: 21512031]

[74]   Eulalio A, Mano M, Dal Ferro M, *et al.* Functional screening identifies miRNAs inducing cardiac regeneration. Nature 2012; 492(7429): 376-81.
[http://dx.doi.org/10.1038/nature11739] [PMID: 23222520]

[75]   Eding J, Van der Spoel T, Vesterinen H, Sena E, Doevendans P, Macleod M, Chamuleau S. Similar effect of autologous and allogeneic cell therapy for ischemic heart disease: results from a meta-analysis of large animal studies. J Am Coll Cardiol 2014; 63(12): A1762.
[http://dx.doi.org/10.1016/S0735-1097(14)61765-4]

[76]   Deb A, Wang S, Skelding KA, Miller D, Simper D, Caplice NM. Bone marrow-derived cardiomyocytes are present in adult human heart: A study of gender-mismatched bone marrow transplantation patients. Circulation 2003; 107(9): 1247-9.
[http://dx.doi.org/10.1161/01.CIR.0000061910.39145.F0] [PMID: 12628942]

[77]   Yacoub MH, Terrovitis J. CADUCEUS, SCIPIO, ALCADIA: Cell therapy trials using cardiac-derived cells for patients with post myocardial infarction LV dysfunction, still evolving. Glob Cardiol Sci Pract 2013; 2013(1): 5-8.
[http://dx.doi.org/10.5339/gcsp.2013.3] [PMID: 24688997]

[78]   Nussbaum J, Minami E, Laflamme MA, *et al.* Transplantation of undifferentiated murine embryonic stem cells in the heart: teratoma formation and immune response. FASEB J 2007; 21(7): 1345-57.
[http://dx.doi.org/10.1096/fj.06-6769com] [PMID: 17284483]

[79]   Min J-Y, Yang Y, Sullivan MF, *et al.* Long-term improvement of cardiac function in rats after infarction by transplantation of embryonic stem cells. J Thorac Cardiovasc Surg 2003; 125(2): 361-9.
[http://dx.doi.org/10.1067/mtc.2003.101] [PMID: 12579106]

[80]   Madden LR, Mortisen DJ, Sussman EM, *et al.* Proangiogenic scaffolds as functional templates for cardiac tissue engineering. Proc Natl Acad Sci USA 2010; 107(34): 15211-6.
[http://dx.doi.org/10.1073/pnas.1006442107] [PMID: 20696917]

[81]   Fisher SA, Brunskill SJ, Doree C, Mathur A, Taggart DP, Martin-Rendon E. Stem cell therapy for chronic ischaemic heart disease and congestive heart failure. Cochrane Database Syst Rev 2014; 4(4)CD007888

[http://dx.doi.org/10.1002/14651858.CD007888.pub2] [PMID: 24777540]

[82]   Xu J, Du Y, Deng H. Direct lineage reprogramming: strategies, mechanisms, and applications. Cell Stem Cell 2015; 16(2): 119-34.
[http://dx.doi.org/10.1016/j.stem.2015.01.013] [PMID: 25658369]

[83]   Ebrahimi B. *In vivo* reprogramming for heart regeneration: A glance at efficiency, environmental impacts, challenges and future directions. J Mol Cell Cardiol 2017; 108: 61-72.
[http://dx.doi.org/10.1016/j.yjmcc.2017.05.005] [PMID: 28502796]

[84]   Chow A, Stuckey DJ, Kidher E, *et al.* Human induced pluripotent stem cell-derived cardiomyocyte encapsulating bioactive hydrogels improve rat heart function post myocardial infarction. Stem Cell Reports 2017; 9(5): 1415-22.
[http://dx.doi.org/10.1016/j.stemcr.2017.09.003] [PMID: 28988988]

[85]   Nguyen MM, Carlini AS, Chien M-P, *et al.* Enzyme-Responsive Nanoparticles for Targeted Accumulation and Prolonged Retention in Heart Tissue after Myocardial Infarction. Adv Mater 2015; 27(37): 5547-52.
[http://dx.doi.org/10.1002/adma.201502003] [PMID: 26305446]

[86]   Whyte W, Roche ET, Varela CE, *et al.* Sustained release of targeted cardiac therapy with a replenishable implanted epicardial reservoir. Nat Biomed Eng 2018; 2(6): 416-28.
[http://dx.doi.org/10.1038/s41551-018-0247-5] [PMID: 31011199]

[87]   Paulis LE, Geelen T, Kuhlmann MT, *et al.* Distribution of lipid-based nanoparticles to infarcted myocardium with potential application for MRI-monitored drug delivery. J Control Release 2012; 162(2): 276-85.
[http://dx.doi.org/10.1016/j.jconrel.2012.06.035] [PMID: 22771978]

[88]   Lundy DJ, Chen KH, Toh EK, Hsieh PCH. Distribution of systemically administered nanoparticles reveals a size-dependent effect immediately following cardiac ischaemia-reperfusion injury. Sci Rep 2016; 6: 25613.
[http://dx.doi.org/10.1038/srep25613] [PMID: 27161857]

[89]   Weis SM. Vascular permeability in cardiovascular disease and cancer. Curr Opin Hematol 2008; 15(3): 243-9.
[http://dx.doi.org/10.1097/MOH.0b013e3282f97d86] [PMID: 18391792]

[90]   van der Meel R, Lammers T, Hennink WE. Cancer nanomedicines: oversold or underappreciated? Expert Opin Drug Deliv 2017; 14(1): 1-5.
[http://dx.doi.org/10.1080/17425247.2017.1262346] [PMID: 27852113]

[91]   Cassani M, Fernandes S, Vrbsky J, Ergir E, Cavalieri F, Forte G. Combining Nanomaterials and Developmental Pathways to Design New Treatments for Cardiac Regeneration: The Pulsing Heart of Advanced Therapies. Front Bioeng Biotechnol 2020; 8: 323.
[http://dx.doi.org/10.3389/fbioe.2020.00323] [PMID: 32391340]

[92]   Ergir E, Bachmann B, Redl H, Forte G, Ertl P. Small force, big impact: next generation organ-on-a-chip systems incorporating biomechanical cues. Front Physiol 2018; 9: 1417.
[http://dx.doi.org/10.3389/fphys.2018.01417] [PMID: 30356887]

[93]   Rothbauer M, Rosser JM, Zirath H, Ertl P. Tomorrow today: organ-on-a-chip advances towards clinically relevant pharmaceutical and medical *in vitro* models. Curr Opin Biotechnol 2019; 55: 81-6.
[http://dx.doi.org/10.1016/j.copbio.2018.08.009] [PMID: 30189349]

CHAPTER 12

Smart Nanomaterials for Cardiac Regeneration Therapy

Ranjita Misra[1] and **Fahima Dilnawaz[2],***

[1] *Centre for Molecular and Nanomedical Sciences, Sathyabama Institute of Science and Technology , Chennai-600119, Tamil Nadu, India*

[2] *Laboratory of Nanomedicine, Institute of Life Sciences, Nalco Square, Chandrasekharpur, Bhubaneswar-751023, Odisha, India*

Abstract: Cardiovascular disease (CVDs) have been observed as the major cause of death worldwide. During the cardiac attack, the blood flow slows down, by which the pumping gets affected. For getting the heart functional, sometimes several surgeries are done that weakens the heart. In ultima cases, loss of heart cells led to a heart attack. The therapeutic options that are adapted for preventing CVDs patients are often being treated with invasive cardiac surgery. Lack of solution to heart troubles and its underlying mechanism led towards the drive of regeneration therapy. Tissue engineering and regenerative strategies goal serves a dual purpose, firstly to stop disease progression and secondly to reverse disease effects to regain and restore heart function. Nanotechnology has been a revolutionary step towards cardiac therapy. Through nanotechnology, there has been a great paradigm shift in the treatment of coronary heart diseases, heart injury, muscle cells improvement, normal functioning of the heart after massive injuries. Tissue-engineered therapeutics are basically delivered to the heart by two approaches, such as cardiac injections and cardiac patches. Engineered nanoparticles for the specific purpose of cardiac ailment play a vital role in heart cure and biomedical application.

Keywords: Biomedical application, Biomaterials, Nanotechnology, Nanomaterials, Tissue engineering.

INTRODUCTION

Cardiovascular disease (CVD) is one of the main causes of disability and death worldwide [1]. CVD accounts for approximately 40% of all human mortality [2]. It has been estimated that about 1.8 million from the UK, 5 million from the US, and around 25 million people worldwide are suffering from cardiovascular diseases.

* **Corresponding author Fahima Dilnawaz:** Laboratory of Nanomedicine, Institute of Life Sciences, Nalco Square, Chandrasekharpur, Bhubaneswar-751023, Odisha, India; Tel: +91-674 – 2304341, 2304283, Fax: 91-674-2300728; E-mail: fahimadilnawaz@gmail.com

Poor prognosis with 12 months of diagnosis leads to 40% mortality thereafter, causing around 10% annual mortality. Annually, in the US and UK, this disease causes an economic burden of more than around $33 billion and £700 million, respectively [3]. CVDs mainly means to a group of pathological syndromes found in blood vessels, cardiac and valvular tissues linked with the heart [4]. Myocardial infarction (MI), atherosclerosis, ischemic cardiomyopathy, coronary heart disease, heart failure, atrial fibrillation, angina pectoris, and endocarditis are the major type of heart diseases found throughout the world population. CVD is primarily characterized by the formation of atherosclerotic lesions in small and medium-sized arteries initially that eventually leading to narrowing of vessels and possibly require revascularization. Mostly, these CVDs occur due to augmented workloads in the lining of the blood vessels and muscles of cardiac tissues [5]. Presently, different approaches, such as the use of b-1 receptor blockers, surgical intervention like Coronary artery bypass graft (CABG) surgery, are some of the treatment options available for CVDs management [6]. However, the use of these approaches is limited up to some extent. Due to the limitations of the present treatment modalities and the poor regeneration capacity of the myocardium or cardiac tissue, researchers have now moved to develop advanced approaches aiming at improving the function of the myocardium. They anticipate that promoting the proliferation of cardiomyocyte and heart regeneration might be a promising approach to combat the CVDs to a great extent.

In this regard, nanotechnology has shown promising efficacy in the field of regenerative medicine both in preclinical and clinical settings for biomedical research applications [7]. Till now, the presently existing synthetic materials are lacking in clinical applications because of their lower biocompatibility and lacking in standard physiological responsiveness. A continuous effort of both bio-engineers and tissue engineers, along with their strong understanding of cardiovascular diseases, has directed the investigators towards developed regenerative strategies, emphasizing new materials for formulating better temporary scaffold-like structures that enhance the self-regeneration of naïve tissues [8]. Mostly, these materials include biocompatible and biodegradable polymers that can synthetically be prepared or occurred naturally. These biopolymers have scaffold-like characteristics that provide a microenvironment resembling the extracellular matrix of native tissues [9]. Among different polymers Poly (lactic-co-glycolic acid) (PLGA) is one of the most commonly used synthetic polymers approved for human use because its byproducts such as lactic acid and glycolic acid can easily be metabolized in humans. PLGA establishes a striking podium equally as a scaffold material for cardiovascular disease grafts or stents and also as a polymeric drug delivery carrier system [10]. Similarly, alginate is an abundantly used natural polymer that has shown promising results clinically. This is highly accepted for various medical applications in humans because of its non-toxic, biocompatibility, non-thrombogenic, and non-immunogenic nature. Alginate-constructed hydrogels offer good mechanical properties and an aqueous atmosphere essential for metabolic exchange, lead to effective pilot clinical trials of alginate-based injectable scaffolds for treating the left ventricular remodeling after myocardial infarction [11]. Thus, in this chapter, we will discuss the CVDs and their treatment by using smart nanomaterials.

FATAL IMPACT OF CARDIOVASCULAR DISEASES (CVD)

Cardiovascular diseases are remained to be the number one cause of death globally. CVD has already been declared as the leading cause of death by the World Health Organization (WHO). CVD usually affects both men and women in equal proportion. It has been estimated by WHO that around 23.6 million people will die by 2030 due to CVD conditions such as stroke and heart disease [12]. Although these circumstances continue predominant in universal mortality rates, people can initiate steps to avoid them. The devastating and regular fatal difficulties of CVDs frequently occur in middle-aged people or elderly men and women [13]. Usually, CVDs refer to a number of conditions as the most prevalent one is heart disease, which is linked to a process known as atherosclerosis. This condition refers to a condition that when a substance known as plaque gets deposited in the walls of the arteries, which leads to the narrowing of the arteries, subsequently blocking the blood flow [14]. Moreover, atherosclerosis mainly leads to the development of coronary, cerebral and peripheral artery disease. It usually begins early in life then progresses slowly to adulthood. It is generally asymptomatic for a long time. The degree of development of atherosclerosis is mostly affected by cardiovascular risk factors like the use of tobacco, sedimental lifestyle and unhealthy diet, high blood pressure, blood lipid, and blood glucose level [15]. Continuous exposure to the mentioned risk factors leads to the formation of plaques, blood vessel narrowing and blockage in blood flow to vital organs such as the brain or heart. This leads to a heart stroke or attack. Maximum individuals stay alive after their first heart attack and lead a normal life living for many more years with productive activity. However, the onset of heart attack does not ask the necessity of changes. The lifestyle changes and medications recommended by the doctor mostly depend on the extent of your heart damage and the degree of heart attack caused by the heart disease. Another type of CVD is an ischemic stroke caused due by blockage of blood supply by the blood vessel to the brain, mostly from a blood clot [16]. Heart failure, sometimes called congestive heart failure, is a type of CVD where the heart will not pump the blood. Arrhythmia is a type of CVDs which is related to the abnormal type of heart rhythm, such as the rhythm can be too slow, too fast or irregular [17]. One more type of CVD is the heart valve problems in which the heart valves do not open or function properly for blood flow through as they should. The total risk of cardiovascular disease risk mainly depends on a particular risk factor of an individual, such as his profile, age and sex. The risk is higher with older people along with other risk factors that for women with lower age and with few risk factors. However, the total risk of progressing CVDs is mainly estimated by the joint effect of different cardiovascular risk factors that coexist and affect manifold. A person with numerous slightly elevated risk factors may be at a developed whole risk of CVD than somebody with just one raised risk factor. These CVDs affect many middle-aged people, extremely affecting their income and savings. CVDs also lead to loss in earnings with the high-cost health care payments that weaken the development of country both socially and economically [18]. Thus, CVDs exhibit a substantial problem on the economies of the nations. Appropriate and continuous lifestyle intrusions and, when required, use of the drug will decrease the danger of CVDs, like heart attacks and strokes. This prevents or reduces the occurrence of premature death, disability and mortality. Most people are not aware of their CVDs risk status, such as high blood pressure, abnormal blood lips, and glucose level. Therefore, these predicted risk factors may be useful to guide people to lower the risk of the onset of CVDs by controlling their lifestyle and changing dietary and physical activity habits.

CURRENT TREATMENT STRATEGIES FOR CVD AND THEIR LIMITATIONS

Despite the countless efforts in the treatment and prevention, cardiovascular diseases are considered as the principal reason for premature death and disability throughout the world. Increased workloads in the lining of blood vessels and in the muscles of the cardiac tissues are the main reason for the occurrence of CVDs. For managing the CVDs, an integrative approach has shown great effect. This integrative approach addresses several of the main causes which are affected by the lifestyle, thus it is preferably suitable for the prevention and treatment of CVDs. There is available a broad spectrum of therapies for CVDs management [19]. Nutrition is possibly the furthermost influential remedy obtainable for the prevention and treatment of CVDs. This has been proved by the outstanding results obtained from the Lyon Diet Heart Study. In this investigation, the myocardial infraction survivor patients were divided into two groups based on their type of uptake of diet. The control group was taking a prudent diet containing reduced cholesterol and total fat. The other group had Mediterranean-style food that consists of food with less oil, more vegetables and fruit. The study showed that daily eating of green leafy vegetables is linked with the 23% reduction of artery diseases [20]. Patients frequently ask about "natural" approaches for the management of cardiovascular diseases. In performance with dietary regulation, regular exercise is one more potent therapy. It has been seen that daily 30 minutes of walking is associated with 18% reduction CVDs chances of occurrence. Moreover, aerobic exercises are generally recommended for cardiovascular health. Additional vigorous exercises of a long time are expected to be of even better effect. Obviously, individual treatments necessary to take into consideration the patient's overall fitness past and cardiovascular status. Stress checking before starting a routine may be suitable for those with a past of heart disease or those with many cardiovascular risk factors, mostly those who have been formerly inactive. In addition to nutrition and exercise as "basics" of heart health, patients with cardiovascular disease should have treated with currently available advanced treatments or technologies. Thus, with the diagnosis of chronic heart failure, the first line of treatment includes the blocking of b1-receptors that are present in the cardiomyocytes cell membrane. The increased pressure on the heart leads to the further secretion of adrenaline because of sympathetic nervous system outflow, subsequently leading to abnormal expression of b1-receptors. This, b1-receptors are controlled by the blockers that competitively bind to block the sympathetic nervous system in the heart. The b-1 blockers help in reducing the contraction of heart muscles and blood vessels which decreases the heart workload [21].

The second-line treatment option for CVDs is a surgical approach that restores the supply of blood to the heart muscle. This surgery is known as coronary artery bypass graft (CABG) surgery that is a critical surgical procedure in which the blocked blood vessels are bridged through native or synthetic grafts. The choice of the graft to be used mainly depends up on the cardiac tissue damage extent. The increased patency and less immunological issues with native grafts have been considered as the gold standard for CABG. The legs, arms, blood vessels, abdomen and chest of the patients itself are served as a source of grafts. Mostly CABG grafts are isolated from thoracic mammary arteries, the saphenous vein of the legs, gastroepiploic artery, and radial arteries of inner forearms [6].

There exist some alternative approaches for CVDs such as bare-metal stents, angioplasty and drug eluting stents. One implant device, such as implantable cardioverter defibrillators (ICD) are available to prevent death even after heart failure caused by ventricular tachycardia. Recent progress in bioelectronics led to the development of next-generation ICDs exhibiting dual functions of a pacemaker or defibrillator. The probes in ICDs can able to detect electrical signal changes aroused due to bradycardia or tachycardia. In ICDs, the electric signals are received and directed to the affected areas with the help of internal batteries and power generators. The ventricular arrhythmias that rise due to myocardial infarction and electrolyte imbalances are mostly corrected by ICDs. However, the ICD implantation in patient's skin may lead to some minor uneasiness. Still, it helps in improving the quality of life [22].

IMPORTANCE OF TISSUE REGENERATION IN CVD

Despite great advances in the management of CVDs, conventional strategies are able to reduce the pathological burden only to a certain extent, however, these cannot repair the damaged myocardial tissues. Recently, the improved therapy strategy used in clinics for controlling the left ventricle (LV) dilation and aneurysm linked to cardiac failure is by using the patches taken from the bovine small intestine or porcine pericardium. This type of patchable to maintain the function of the heart by acting as a physical barrier, thereby preventing the further thinning of the left ventricle. However, the *in vivo* application of such patches face challenges due to xenogeneic origin and biodegradability issues [23]. Present treatment strategies are still limited for cardiovascular diseases, especially for atherosclerosis and myocardial infarction. With the presently available treatment, the dead cells formed due to acute myocardial infarction (MI) are cannot be replaced or regenerated with stem cell recruitment. Moreover, the rate of loss of cardiomyocytes is very higher than the self-renewal of the stem cells. Thus, at the region of infract non-contractile scar tissue forms that lead to the loss of myocardial contractile function subsequently to congestive heart failure [24]. Traditionally, biological (auto or allografts) or mechanical valves were implanted for heart disease, however, this is limited by the smaller number of donors that cannot meet the demand of an increased number of patients that require treatment. In this regard, engineered cardiac tissue or stem cells construction evolved as a promising approach towards CVDs management [25]. For example, previously, Li *et al.* have cultured foetal rat myocytes on gelatin meshes [26]. One week later, meshes were fixed into the myocardial scar tissue or subcutaneous tissue of a cryoinjured rat heart. After 5 weeks, regular and spontaneous contraction of the grafts in subcutaneous tissue was found. Whereas the survival and formation of junctions were observed in myocardial scar tissue graft. The final goal of engineered cardiac tissues (ECTs) is to recreate a model from the injured cardiac tissues with intact and original structure and function. The graft requires to have several properties such as (1) enhancement in the growth and differentiation of stem cells, (2) should be biocompatible, and (3) adequate elasticity (tension and compressive) in order to lessen the chances of arrhythmias or dysfunctions.

NANOTECHNOLOGY AND CARDIAC TISSUE REGENERATION

The speedy progress of nanotechnology through the past ten years has led to novel viewpoints and developments in biomedical research and also in clinical practice. As nanotechnology is well-defined by the size of a material (usually 1–100 nm) or handling at the molecular level, it includes a wide variety of nanoscale materials used in numerous areas of regenerative medicine, such as cell therapy, diagnosis, drug/gene delivery and tissue engineering (TE) [27]. Thus, the use of nanotechnology is widely spread almost in all aspects of biomedicine, from biomimetic engineered scaffold and drug delivery systems to biosensors [28]. In the context of tissue engineering polymers and biomaterials are processed to nanometer range and can be aggregated and organized in an ordered manner to get three-dimensional tissues and organs [29]. Conventionally, auto- and allo-grafts (top-down approach) were used to rebuild tissue function after damage or injury of the organs or tissues. Alternatively, nanomaterials in a bottom-up approach offer an organized way of tissues or organ construction. These nanomaterials can be used as a scaffold or as drug delivery carriers for the delivery of drugs to the disease site that is limited with the necessary regulators for cell migration, re-growth, or differentiation [30]. The fundamental step in tissue engineering is the creation of biocompatible scaffolds containing live cells and/or therapeutic/bioactive molecules that can repair or regenerate the damaged cells or tissues. The vital characteristics of an ideal scaffold include appropriate physical properties for better attachment of cells or tissues for proper cell proliferation, precise porosity and permeability and biocompatibility. Moreover, the bioadhesive properties of the biomaterials are improved with the supplement of nanotopographies to achieve better cell adhesion and growth. Such as surface roughness is a good example that influences the cell attachment and growth spreading. Furthermore, the large surface area of nanomaterials improves the cell-surface interactions by increasing the adsorption of surface adhesive proteins such as vitronectin and fibronectin that bind to cells through integrins [31]. Therefore, the advancement in nanotechnology has led researchers to formulate scaffolds having characteristics physical properties that affect the biological activity of the cells or tissues and also mimic the natural cell environment. So far, the function of infracted myocardial heart has been improved *in vitro* by using contractile cardiac grafts. Moreover, the faulty heart valves function has also improved with the injection of nanomaterials in heart valve tissue engineering that has emerged as alternatives for improved valvular heart surgery [32].

Presently, both natural or synthetic scaffolds have been exploited in order to develop a valuable scaffold clinically for a particular tissue or organ [33]. Clinically applied natural scaffolds include decellularized dermis or xenogeneic vessels for treating burn injuries and vascular function restoration, respectively [34]. These scaffolds have exhibited potential results in tissue repair, but still, they lack with strong mechanical strength, degradability, immunogenic and cross-contamination. Conversely, synthetic or combination of synthetic and natural polymers have shown effective results in tissue repairing. The commonly used natural polymers include alginate, collagen, basement membrane, hyaluronan, agarose and demineralized bone matrix [35]. Synthetic polymers comprise biodegradable polymers such as poly (D, L-lactide-co-glycolide) (PLGA), polyglycolic acid (PGA), *etc* [36]. These polymers are well established for clinical use and are presently also used in many tissue engineering applications. The development of nanofibrous scaffold prepared by electrospinning technique is assumed to be a feasible method for producing cardiac grafts with clinically applicable features. A number of biomaterials have been used alone or in combination in order to achieve the necessities of cardiac regeneration. The primary aim to find the polymers with proper elasticity and mechanical properties which can mimic the required features of cardiac tissue. In this context, properly oriented combination of PCL and gelatin yield outstanding results thereby improving the adhesion and alignment of myocardial cells in the nanofibrous scaffold. In a recent study, it has been investigated that nanofibrous scaffolds composed of L-lactic acid with trimethylene carbonate (P(L)LA-*co*-TMC) help in enhanced proliferation of cardiomyocytes and proficiently reserves the cell surface topography, without hindering the actin marker expression, thus representing its potent effect for myocardial tissue engineering [37]. Additionally, a current investigation discovered the suitable proportion of poly(1,8-octanediol-*co*-citrate) (POC) and poly(L-lactic acid)-*co*-poly--3-caprolactone) (PLCL) to attain a nanosized scaffold with proper elasticity and tensile strength, comparable to cardiac tissue [38]. Furthermore, scientists have established a biocompatible scaffold with multiple activities such as good physicochemical and mechanical features and also is capable of differentiating cells into cardiomyocytes. Thus, Gupta *et al.* have developed a scaffold comprising PEG-PCL-CPCL loaded with a bone morphogenetic protein (BMP) that helps in the differentiation of embryonic stem cells toward functional cardiomyocytes [39]. Moreover, Sreerekha *et al.* demonstrated a scaffold made up of PLGA and fibrin is capable of promoting cardiomyocyte MSC differentiation [40]. Similarly, investigations have formulated a fibronectin-coated chitosan nano scaffold with co-culture of cardiomyocyte-fibroblast which provides a structure similar to cardiac tissue where the cardiomyocytes preserved their morphology and synchronously contracted [41]. Newly, PEG nanoscaffold embedded in fibrin hydrogel in combination with cardiac progenitor cells have used as cardiac patches, that were fixed in the wall of the ventricle of a rat myocardial infarction model. The implanted patch growths the infracted area with augmented cell viability and ECM collagen organization [42]. Further nanotechnological variant comprises using NPs, that show significant benefits for a targeted treatment. For example, NPs can effortlessly cross the endothelial lining, and can be delivered by a non-invasive technique, intravenously or by inhalation. Abundant *in vivo* investigations have demonstrated the rewards of using NPs as complementary therapy for cardiovascular diseases. For instance, phosphatidylserine liposomes delivered *via* intravenous route into a mouse with myocardial infarction, showed helping angiogenesis, remodelling and to stop ventricular dilatation. Furthermore, NPs have been used to permit factor and/or cytokine delivery [7, 43].

SMART NANOMATERIALS: EMERGING APPROACH IN REGENERATION THERAPY

Although TE approach promises better therapeutic regime, still it faces numerous limitations; hence transcribing these ideas into reality seems like an uphill task. Because most of the time the engineered materials inability to mimic the natural properties of tissues becomes the roadblock. With the help of nanotechnology different types of smart nanomaterials (metallic, non-metallic, polymeric as shown in Fig. **1**) can be synthesized towards more complex and efficient nanofibers and nanopatterned surfaces for better cell behavior in TEM as well as providing mechanical strength and controlled release of bioactive agents [44]. Metallic nanoparticles such as gold and silver nanoparticles showcasing the conducting and antimicrobial properties and also the fluorescence properties of the quantum dots as well as electromechanical properties of carbon nanotubes (CNTs) are beneficial in numerous TE applications.

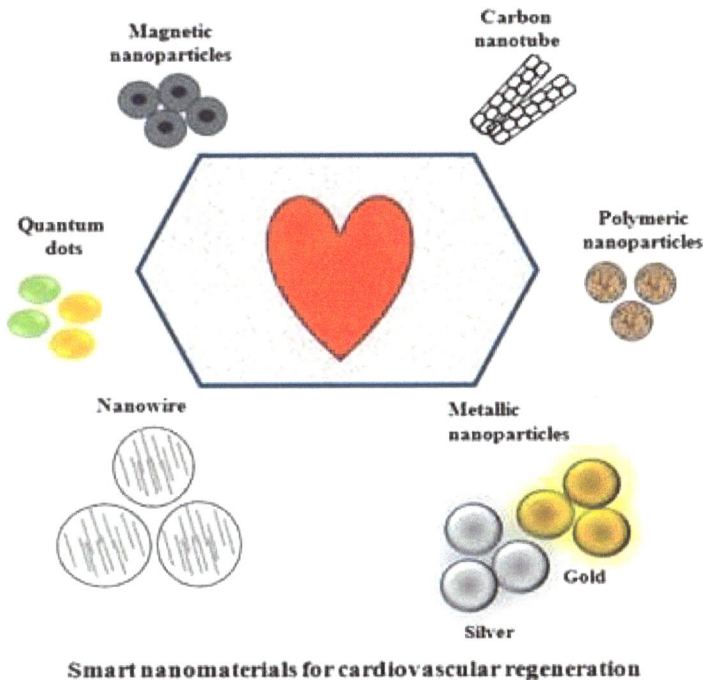

Smart nanomaterials for cardiovascular regeneration

Fig. (1). Metallic, non-metallic and polymeric smart nanoparticles are used for cardiovascular regeneration.

In the study of cell mechano-transduction, gene delivery, controlling cell patterning and construction of complex 3D tissues, magnetic nanoparticles (MNPs) are widely used. Izadifar *et al.*, developed bilayer polymeric nanoparticles which was featured for low burst effect and time-delayed release, and allowed for sequential release of platelet-derived growth factor (PDGF) following co-release of vascular endothelial growth factor (VEGF) and basic fibroblast growth factor (bFGF), for cardiac tissue engineering for myocardial infarction repair by promoting angiogenesis [45]. Myocardial infarction is the most common cause of heart failure, current therapies makes the progression of heart failure sluggish, but unable to tackle the progressive loss of cardiomyocytes after heart attack [46]. In this regard, implantable constructs (*e.g.,* cardiac patches) through cardiac tissue engineering would provide physical and biochemical cues allowing for myocardium regeneration [47, 48]. Therefore, spatiotemporal control of growth factor (GF) release is paramount but remains unachievable. So, development of smart polymeric particulate delivery systems enables improvements over the control of GF. This angiogenic factor-loaded were biologically active PLGA polymeric nanoparticles can significantly stimulated endothelial sprouting angiogenesis in the nanoparticle-incorporated fibrin matrix, by which The angiogenesis was improved compared to control [45].Further for better functionality *in vivo*, Izadifar *et al.*, also developed a Geno-Neural model consisting of a trained artificial neural network (ANN) coupled with genetic algorithm (GA) for the prediction and optimum combinations of multiple physical and polymeric variables of the nanoparticles to achieve a predetermined release pattern(s). As an example, a cardiac patch implanted on an infarction area that is which lacks blood vessels should be able to direct angiogenesis from the patch circumference, which is in close contact with the healthy tissue, to the patch centre, located near the infarction. To sustainably direct angiogenesis sprouts from preexisting vessels at the patch boundary toward the centre requires the establishment of a VEGF gradient from the patch boundaries toward the centre [49]. A vascularization strategy demands a rate-programmable delivery system to synchronize VEGF gradient and angiogenesis using the Geno-Neural model would allow the nanoparticles to be precisely laid down along with a printable hydrogel in a cardiac patch using 3D-bioplotting technology [45] to achieve spatiotemporal control of GF release in the cardiac patch. Hydrogel nanoparticulate system is a network of polymer chains that are composed of hydrophilic polymers. Cardiovascular regenerative medicine using hydrogels combined with cells, can be directly injected into the cardiac damaged areas to enhance the cardiac differentiation and initiate electrophysiological maturation of the 3-dimensional (3D) structure of the heart following MI [50]. In a study, injection of a non-degradable polyethylene glycol (PEG) gel in a rat infarction model resulted in significant permeation of macrophages, suggesting an immune response [51]. In another study Duan and his colleagues developed bioinks which has high viscosity and low stiffness for 3D printing of organs or patches. This was made skillfully by deploying the relative amounts of methacrylated hyaluronic acid and methacrylated gelatin which can result in improved cell spreading and fibroblastic phenotype maintenance. In this hybrid hydrogel human aortic valvular interstitial cells (HAVICs) were encapsulated, where 3D trileaflet valves were channeled with HAVICs. Post seven days of culture, the encapsulated HAVICs displayed better cell viability and appropriate cell-type morphologies which could express all target genes like, vimentin, periostin, collagen and α-smooth muscle actin (αSMA) [52]. For the enhancement of growth, differentiation, or physiological function the hydrogels could be functionalized with small molecules, peptides, or proteins. For myocardial therapy, Paul *et al*, developed injectable and biocompatible hydrogel by which a nanocomplex of graphene oxide (GO) and vascular endothelial growth factor-165 (VEGF) pro-angiogenic gene can be efficiently delivered. This localized genetherapy was achieved by nonviral gene delivery vehicle made from polyethylenimine (PEI) functionalized GO nanosheets (fGO), later complexed with DNA-VEGF and incorporated in the low-modulus methacrylated gelatin (GelMA) hydrogel. Hydrogel nanocomposites could efficiently transfect myocardial tissues and induced favorable therapeutic effects without raising any cytotoxic effects [53]. Godier-Furnémont *et al*, established tissue engineering platform with a fully biological composite scaffold for the delivery of human mesenchymal progenitor cells (MPCs). This biological composite scaffold was preconditioned with MPC, for formation of greater vascular network in the infarct bed by the secretion of paracrine factors (SDF-1), that directed the migration of MPCs into ischemic myocardium, but not on normal myocardium [54]. Another myocardial-specific hydrogel, was derived from decellularized ventricular ECM, developed which can self-assembles when injected *in vivo*. With these injected endogenous cardiomyocytes was increased in the infarct area and inturn maintains cardiac function without inducing arrhythmias [55]. For 3-D bioprinting, Jia *et al.*, utilized oxidised alginate-based bioink for tissue-specific tissue engineering applications. In which four alginate solutions with varied biodegradability were printed with human adipose-derived stem cells (hADSCs) into lattice-structure, these cell-laden hydrogels eventually with high accuracy modulated proliferation and spreading of hADSCs without affecting the structure integrity of the lattice structures after 8 days in culture [56]. Direct differentiation of pluripotent cardioprogenitors, using P19 embryonal carcinoma (EC) cells were precisely controlled by using synthetic three-dimensional (3D) matrix metalloproteinase (MMP)-sensitive poly (ethylene glycol) (PEG)-based hydrogels. It served as an alternative to natural matrices for engineering cardiac tissue structures for cell culture and further potential therapeutic applications [57]. In another study, for an effective delivery alginate hydrogel was used for intracoronary injection into the infarcted myocardium to prevent left ventricular (LV) remodeling early after myocardial infarction (MI).

Post injected harvested hearts displayed that alginate hydrogel have crossed and deposited in the infarcted leaky vessels suggesting an improvement to repair MI [58].

Cardiac stem cells (CSCs) based therapy is an emerging aspect for ischemic cardiomyopathy. In a study CSC was encapsulated within matrix-enriched hydrogel capsules for better cell survival, post-ischemic cell retention and cardiac function. Encapsulated stem cells promoted acute retention of CSCs and repaired infarcted myocardium by preventing mechanical clearance from the heart while protecting against anoikis [59]. Karoubi *et al*, used single-cell hydrogel capsule for the enhancement of cell survival of adherent cells in transient suspension culture. To promote cell-matrix survival signals, in an agarose capsules human marrow stromal cells (hMSCs) were singularly encapsulated containing the immobilized matrix molecules, fibronectin and fibrinogen. These encapsulated hMSCs demonstrated augmented viability, better metabolic activity and improved cell-cytoskeletal patterning by re-induction of cell-matrix interactions likely *via* integrin clustering and subsequent activation of the extracellular signaling cascade of MAPK (ERK)/mitogen activated protein kinase (MAPK) [60]. Cheng *et al*, used iron-labeled cardiosphere-derived cells in MI for the improvement of engraftment and functional benefit. Cardiosphere-derived cells (CDCs) labelled with magnetic nanoparticles were injected intramyocardially. With aid of external magnet cells were visibly attracted towards the magnetic zone and accumulated around the ischemic region, whereas the nontargeted cells were washed out immediately after injection. With magnetic targeting cell retention, engraftment, functional benefit could be improved [61].

FUTURE PERSPECTIVE OF CARDIAC CLINICAL THERAPY

Damaged myocardium is known for its incapability to regenerate. Stem cell therapy for MI in most cases is attributed to the reduction of myocardial necrosis following ischemic injury. Recently a technique is developed with pericardium-derived de novo cardiomyocytes to induce myocardial regeneration with increased vascularity [62]. Epicardial cells derived de novo regenerated myocardium was beneficial. With autologous adipose-derived stem cell (AdSC) therapy for ischemic heart diseases (IHDs) clinical trials are ongoing. Yokoyama *et al.*, recently attempted combinational therapeutic formulation of nanoparticles using poly(lactic-co-glycolic) acid (PLGA) loaded with AdSCs and simvastatin for spontaneous cardiac regeneration in ischemic myocardium, displaying the recovery of impaired cardiac function. Simvastatin-conjugated nanoparticles (SimNPs) significantly promoted migration, improved cardiac function by inducing endogenous cardiac regeneration. Direct recruited AdSCs can contribute to tissue regeneration as novel somatic stem cell therapy for ischemic heart disease. For potential clinical application mesenchymal stem cell (MSC) therapy are sought, but it lacks poor engraftment. However, to make it clinically useful alternative cell-free therapy using MSC-derived exosomes have emerged for treatment of MI. However, following injection diffusion of exosomes out of the infarcted heart displays low productivity which limits its potential clinical applications. Lee *et al*, developed and utilized exosome-mimetic extracellular nanovesicles (NVs) derived from iron oxide nanoparticles (IONPs)–incorporated MSCs (IONP-MSCs) to an infarcted myocardium. Post injection the retention of IONP-NVs in the infarcted myocardium was greatly enhanced with external application of magnetic field for 24 hours. It also exhibited reduced infarct size, decreased apoptosis, inflammation, as well as improved angiogenesis and cardiac function recovery [63]. Vandergriff *et al*, used human cardiosphere-derived stem cells (hCDCs) were labelled with FDA-approved ferumoxytol nanoparticles Feraheme® (F) in the presence of heparin (H) and protamine (P) for intracoronarily infusion into syngeneic rats. Magnetic targeting enables increase of acute cell retention towards more attenuated left ventricular remodeling and greater therapeutic benefit (ejection fraction) 3 weeks after treatment [64]. Cheng *et al*, used application of magnetic field for the retention improvement of retention of rat cardiosphere-derived cells by preventing venous washout after post injection into the rat heart with open chest myocardial infarction [61]. For the improvement of electrical communication between adjacent cardiac cells, gold nanowire cardiac patches were developed using alginate scaffolds which can bridge the electrically resistant pore walls with the help of alginate. After electrical stimulation tissues grown on these composite matrices were thicker and better aligned and contracted synchronously than that of those grown on pristine alginate. Further through cardiac tissue engineering process myocardial infarction can be treated by using 3D biomaterials based cardiac patches to which contracting cells can be seed in or onto before transplantation [65]. A 3D hybrid nanocomposite hydrogel scaffold was developed by which online monitoring and regulation of tissue function can be studied by integrating flexible cardiac cells with freestanding electronics which in turn enables the recording of cellular electrical activities and synchronization of cell contraction. Complex electronics integration within cardiac patches will eventually provide therapeutic control and regulation of cardiac function [66].

CONCLUSION

Cardiovascular diseases remain the major cause of death globally, despite of people's welcoming healthier life styles according to WHO, 2019. Cardiac therapy research is challenged by the limited inherent regenerative capacity of the adult heart. Novel strategies to promote cardiac regeneration lags behind. In this regard, development of new therapies are sought which can induce cardiac protection and repair and eventually improving the life quality of the patient. Nanoparticles unique features has been extensively exploited to overcome the limitations of standard medical therapies. According to the need currently, nanoparticles can be tuned and designed opportunely for specific cardiac applications. To enhance the therapeutics delivery, innovative biomaterials and strategies of investigation of new pathways to be studied to reach cardiac homeostasis. Further integration of living cells and electronic function by fusing it with multifunctional electronics and engineered cardiac patches (where living cells and tissues interact with electronics to improve tissue function) represents a new route in tissue engineering where clinicians can be notified regarding the progress patient's health condition. In order to bring potential therapeutic nanomedical devices for cardiac regeneration closer association of nanotechnologist together with cell and molecular biologists and clinicians can led to fruitful clinical translation.

CONSENT FOR PUBLICATION

Not Applicable.

CONFLICT OF INTEREST

The author confirms that this chapter contents have no conflict of interest.

ACKNOWLEDGEMENT

FD gratefully acknowledges Dept. of Science and Technology, Govt. of India, for the financial grant [SR/WOS-A/LS-448/2017(G)] in the form of women scientist fellowship (WOS-A).

REFERENCES

[1]   Authors/Task Force Members; ESC Committee for Practice Guidelines (CPG); ESC National Cardiac Societies. 2019 ESC/EAS guidelines for the management of dyslipidaemias: Lipid modification to reduce cardiovascular risk. Atherosclerosis 2019; 290: 140-205.
[http://dx.doi.org/10.1016/j.atherosclerosis.2019.08.014] [PMID: 31591002]

[2]   Jokinen E. Obesity and cardiovascular disease. Minerva Pediatr 2015; 67(1): 25-32.
[PMID: 25387321]

[3]   Gaziano TA. Cardiovascular disease in the developing world and its cost-effective management. Circulation 2005; 112(23): 3547-53.
[http://dx.doi.org/10.1161/CIRCULATIONAHA.105.591792] [PMID: 16330695]

[4]   Leong DP, Joseph PG, McKee M, *et al.* Reducing the Global Burden of Cardiovascular Disease, Part 2: Prevention and Treatment of Cardiovascular Disease. Circ Res 2017; 121(6): 695-710.
[http://dx.doi.org/10.1161/CIRCRESAHA.117.311849] [PMID: 28860319]

[5]   Van Camp G. Cardiovascular disease prevention. Acta Clin Belg 2014; 69(6): 407-11.
[http://dx.doi.org/10.1179/2295333714Y.0000000069] [PMID: 25176558]

[6]   Velazquez EJ, Lee KL, Jones RH, *et al.* Coronary-Artery Bypass Surgery in Patients with Ischemic Cardiomyopathy. N Engl J Med 2016; 374(16): 1511-20.
[http://dx.doi.org/10.1056/NEJMoa1602001] [PMID: 27040723]

[7]   Prajnamitra RP, Chen HC, Lin CJ, Chen LL, Hsieh PC. Nanotechnology Approaches in Tackling Cardiovascular Diseases. Molecules 2019; 24(10): E2017.
[http://dx.doi.org/10.3390/molecules24102017] [PMID: 31137787]

[8]   Vaidya B, Gupta V. Novel Therapeutic Strategies for Cardiovascular Disease Treatment: From Molecular Level to Nanotechnology. Curr Pharm Des 2015; 21(30): 4367-9.
[http://dx.doi.org/10.2174/1381612821999150917100529] [PMID: 26377649]

[9]   Cooke JP, Atkins J. Nanotherapeutic Solutions for Cardiovascular Disease. Methodist DeBakey Cardiovasc J 2016; 12(3): 132-3.
[http://dx.doi.org/10.14797/mdcj-12-3-132] [PMID: 27826365]

[10]   Danhier F, Ansorena E, Silva JM, Coco R, Le Breton A, Preat V. PLGA-based nanoparticles: an overview of biomedical applications. Journal of controlled release : official journal of the Controlled Release Society 2012; 161(2): 505-22.

[11]   Paul A, Shum-Tim D, Prakash S. Angiogenic nanodelivery systems for myocardial therapy. Methods Mol Biol 2013; 1036: 137-49.
[http://dx.doi.org/10.1007/978-1-62703-511-8_12] [PMID: 23807793]

[12]   Balakumar P, Maung UK, Jagadeesh G. Prevalence and prevention of cardiovascular disease and diabetes mellitus 2016.
[http://dx.doi.org/10.1016/j.phrs.2016.09.040]

[13]   Steptoe A, Kivimäki M. Stress and cardiovascular disease. Nat Rev Cardiol 2012; 9(6): 360-70.
[http://dx.doi.org/10.1038/nrcardio.2012.45] [PMID: 22473079]

[14]   Shoenfeld Y, Sherer Y, Harats D. Artherosclerosis as an infectious, inflammatory and autoimmune disease. Trends Immunol 2001; 22(6): 293-5.
[http://dx.doi.org/10.1016/S1471-4906(01)01922-6] [PMID: 11419409]

[15]   Saar A, Läll K, Alver M, *et al.* Estimating the performance of three cardiovascular disease risk scores: the Estonian Biobank cohort study. J Epidemiol Community Health 2019; 73(3): 272-7.
[http://dx.doi.org/10.1136/jech-2017-209965] [PMID: 30635435]

[16]   Randolph SA. Ischemic Stroke. Workplace Health Saf 2016; 64(9): 444.
[http://dx.doi.org/10.1177/2165079916665400] [PMID: 27621261]

[17]   Biffi A, Rea F, Scotti L, *et al.* Antidepressants and the risk of arrhythmia in elderly affected by a previous cardiovascular disease: a real-life investigation from Italy. Eur J Clin Pharmacol 2018; 74(1): 119-29.
[http://dx.doi.org/10.1007/s00228-017-2352-x] [PMID: 29046942]

[18]   Smith MA. Cardiovascular Disease Update: Foreword. FP Essent 2017; 454: 2.
[PMID: 28266822]

[19]   Aggarwal M, Aggarwal B, Rao J. Integrative Medicine for Cardiovascular Disease and Prevention. Med Clin North Am 2017; 101(5): 895-923.
[http://dx.doi.org/10.1016/j.mcna.2017.04.007] [PMID: 28802470]

[20]   Mozaffarian D. Dietary and Policy Priorities for Cardiovascular Disease, Diabetes, and Obesity: A Comprehensive Review. Circulation 2016; 133(2): 187-225.
[http://dx.doi.org/10.1161/CIRCULATIONAHA.115.018585] [PMID: 26746178]

[21]   Williams MA, Haskell WL, Ades PA, *et al.* Resistance exercise in individuals with and without cardiovascular disease: 2007 update: a scientific statement from the American Heart Association Council on Clinical Cardiology and Council on Nutrition, Physical Activity, and Metabolism. Circulation 2007; 116(5): 572-84.

[http://dx.doi.org/10.1161/CIRCULATIONAHA.107.185214] [PMID: 17638929]

[22] Kodera S, Kiyosue A, Ando J, *et al.* Cost-Effectiveness Analysis of Cardiovascular Disease Treatment in Japan. Int Heart J 2017; 58(6): 847-52.
[http://dx.doi.org/10.1536/ihj.17-365] [PMID: 29151496]

[23] Laflamme MA, Murry CE. Heart regeneration. Nature 2011; 473(7347): 326-35.
[http://dx.doi.org/10.1038/nature10147] [PMID: 21593865]

[24] Galdos FX, Guo Y, Paige SL, VanDusen NJ, Wu SM, Pu WT. Cardiac Regeneration: Lessons From Development. Circ Res 2017; 120(6): 941-59.
[http://dx.doi.org/10.1161/CIRCRESAHA.116.309040] [PMID: 28302741]

[25] Yester JW, Kühn B. Mechanisms of Cardiomyocyte Proliferation and Differentiation in Development and Regeneration. Curr Cardiol Rep 2017; 19(2): 13.
[http://dx.doi.org/10.1007/s11886-017-0826-1] [PMID: 28185170]

[26] Li RK, Jia ZQ, Weisel RD, Mickle DA, Choi A, Yau TM. Survival and function of bioengineered cardiac grafts. Circulation 1999; 100(19) (Suppl.): II63-9.
[http://dx.doi.org/10.1161/01.CIR.100.suppl_2.II-63] [PMID: 10567280]

[27] Misra R, Acharya S, Sahoo SK. Cancer nanotechnology: application of nanotechnology in cancer therapy. Drug Discov Today 2010; 15(19-20): 842-50.
[http://dx.doi.org/10.1016/j.drudis.2010.08.006] [PMID: 20727417]

[28] Parveen S, Misra R, Sahoo SK. Nanoparticles: a boon to drug delivery, therapeutics, diagnostics and imaging. Nanomedicine (Lond) 2012; 8(2): 147-66.
[http://dx.doi.org/10.1016/j.nano.2011.05.016] [PMID: 21703993]

[29] Dunn DA, Hodge AJ, Lipke EA. Biomimetic materials design for cardiac tissue regeneration. Wiley Interdiscip Rev Nanomed Nanobiotechnol 2014; 6(1): 15-39.
[http://dx.doi.org/10.1002/wnan.1241] [PMID: 24123919]

[30] Dilnawaz F, Acharya S, Sahoo SK. Recent trends of nanomedicinal approaches in clinics. Int J Pharm 2018; 538(1-2): 263-78.
[http://dx.doi.org/10.1016/j.ijpharm.2018.01.016] [PMID: 29339248]

[31] Passaro F, Testa G, Ambrosone L, *et al.* Nanotechnology-Based Cardiac Targeting and Direct Cardiac Reprogramming: The Betrothed. Stem Cells Int 2017; 2017: 4940397.
[http://dx.doi.org/10.1155/2017/4940397] [PMID: 29375623]

[32] Radhakrishnan J, Krishnan UM, Sethuraman S. Hydrogel based injectable scaffolds for cardiac tissue regeneration. Biotechnol Adv 2014; 32(2): 449-61.
[http://dx.doi.org/10.1016/j.biotechadv.2013.12.010] [PMID: 24406815]

[33] Lee J, Manoharan V, Cheung L, *et al.* Nanoparticle-Based Hybrid Scaffolds for Deciphering the Role of Multimodal Cues in Cardiac Tissue Engineering. ACS Nano 2019; 13(11): 12525-39.
[http://dx.doi.org/10.1021/acsnano.9b03050] [PMID: 31621284]

[34] Alarçin E, Guan X, Kashaf SS, *et al.* Recreating composition, structure, functionalities of tissues at nanoscale for regenerative medicine. Regen Med 2016; 11(8): 849-58.
[http://dx.doi.org/10.2217/rme-2016-0120] [PMID: 27885900]

[35] G N, Tan A, Gundogan B, *et al.* Tissue engineering vascular grafts a fortiori: looking back and going forward. Expert Opin Biol Ther 2015; 15(2): 231-44.
[http://dx.doi.org/10.1517/14712598.2015.980234] [PMID: 25427995]

[36] Misra R, Acharya S, Dilnawaz F, Sahoo SK. Sustained antibacterial activity of doxycycline-loaded poly(D,L-lactide-co-glycolide) and poly(epsilon-caprolactone) nanoparticles. Nanomedicine (Lond) 2009; 4(5): 519-30.
[http://dx.doi.org/10.2217/nnm.09.28] [PMID: 19572818]

[37] Prabhakaran MP, Mobarakeh LG, Kai D, Karbalaie K, Nasr-Esfahani MH, Ramakrishna S.

Differentiation of embryonic stem cells to cardiomyocytes on electrospun nanofibrous substrates. J Biomed Mater Res B Appl Biomater 2014; 102(3): 447-54.
[http://dx.doi.org/10.1002/jbm.b.33022] [PMID: 24039141]

[38]   Prabhakaran MP, Nair AS, Kai D, Ramakrishna S. Electrospun composite scaffolds containing poly(octanediol-co-citrate) for cardiac tissue engineering. Biopolymers 2012; 97(7): 529-38.
[http://dx.doi.org/10.1002/bip.22035] [PMID: 22328272]

[39]   Gupta V, Lyne DV, Barragan M, Berkland CJ, Detamore MS. Microsphere-based scaffolds encapsulating tricalcium phosphate and hydroxyapatite for bone regeneration. J Mater Sci Mater Med 2016; 27(7): 121.
[http://dx.doi.org/10.1007/s10856-016-5734-1] [PMID: 27272903]

[40]   Sreerekha PR, Menon D, Nair SV, Chennazhi KP. Fabrication of electrospun poly (lactide-c--glycolide)-fibrin multiscale scaffold for myocardial regeneration *in vitro*. Tissue Eng Part A 2013; 19(7-8): 849-59.
[http://dx.doi.org/10.1089/ten.tea.2012.0374] [PMID: 23083104]

[41]   Hussain A, Collins G, Yip D, Cho CH. Functional 3-D cardiac co-culture model using bioactive chitosan nanofiber scaffolds. Biotechnol Bioeng 2013; 110(2): 637-47.
[http://dx.doi.org/10.1002/bit.24727] [PMID: 22991229]

[42]   Geuss LR, Allen AC, Ramamoorthy D, Suggs LJ. Maintenance of HL-1 cardiomyocyte functional activity in PEGylated fibrin gels. Biotechnol Bioeng 2015; 112(7): 1446-56.
[http://dx.doi.org/10.1002/bit.25553] [PMID: 25657056]

[43]   Guo HH, Feng CL, Zhang WX, *et al.* Liver-target nanotechnology facilitates berberine to ameliorate cardio-metabolic diseases. Nat Commun 2019; 10(1): 1981.
[http://dx.doi.org/10.1038/s41467-019-09852-0] [PMID: 31040273]

[44]   Jiang W, Rutherford D, Vuong T, Liu H. Nanomaterials for treating cardiovascular diseases: A review. Bioact Mater 2017; 2(4): 185-98.
[http://dx.doi.org/10.1016/j.bioactmat.2017.11.002] [PMID: 29744429]

[45]   Izadifar M, Kelly ME, Chen X. Regulation of sequential release of growth factors using bilayer polymeric nanoparticles for cardiac tissue engineering. Nanomedicine (Lond) 2016; 11(24): 3237-59.
[http://dx.doi.org/10.2217/nnm-2016-0220] [PMID: 27854552]

[46]   Morice M-CSP, Serruys PW, Kappetein AP, *et al.* Outcomes in patients with de novo left main disease treated with either percutaneous coronary intervention using paclitaxel-eluting stents or coronary artery bypass graft treatment in the Synergy Between Percutaneous Coronary Intervention with TAXUS and Cardiac Surgery (SYNTAX) trial. Circulation 2010; 121(24): 2645-53.
[http://dx.doi.org/10.1161/CIRCULATIONAHA.109.899211] [PMID: 20530001]

[47]   Feng X, Tonnesen MG, Mousa SA, Clark RA. Fibrin and collagen differentially but synergistically regulate sprout angiogenesis of human dermal microvascular endothelial cells in 3-dimensional matrix. Int J Cell Biol 2013; 2013: 231279.
[http://dx.doi.org/10.1155/2013/231279] [PMID: 23737792]

[48]   Guyette JPCJ, Charest JM, Mills RW, *et al.* Bioengineering human myocardium on native extracellular matrix. Circ Res 2016; 118(1): 56-72.
[http://dx.doi.org/10.1161/CIRCRESAHA.115.306874] [PMID: 26503464]

[49]   Izadifar M, Haddadi A, Chen X, Kelly ME. Rate-programming of nano-particulate delivery systems for smart bioactive scaffolds in tissue engineering. Nanotechnology 2015; 26(1): 012001.
[http://dx.doi.org/10.1088/0957-4484/26/1/012001] [PMID: 25474543]

[50]   Vunjak-Novakovic G, Lui KO, Tandon N, Chien KR. Bioengineering heart muscle: a paradigm for regenerative medicine. Annu Rev Biomed Eng 2011; 13: 245-67.
[http://dx.doi.org/10.1146/annurev-bioeng-071910-124701] [PMID: 21568715]

[51]   Dobner S, Bezuidenhout D, Govender P, Zilla P, Davies N. A synthetic non-degradable polyethylene

glycol hydrogel retards adverse post-infarct left ventricular remodeling. J Card Fail 2009; 15(7): 629-36.
[http://dx.doi.org/10.1016/j.cardfail.2009.03.003] [PMID: 19700140]

[52]   Duan Y, Liu Z, O'Neill J, Wan LQ, Freytes DO, Vunjak-Novakovic G. Hybrid gel composed of native heart matrix and collagen induces cardiac differentiation of human embryonic stem cells without supplemental growth factors. J Cardiovasc Transl Res 2011; 4(5): 605-15.
[http://dx.doi.org/10.1007/s12265-011-9304-0] [PMID: 21744185]

[53]   Paul A, Hasan A, Kindi HA, *et al.* Injectable graphene oxide/hydrogel-based angiogenic gene delivery system for vasculogenesis and cardiac repair. ACS Nano 2014; 8(8): 8050-62.
[http://dx.doi.org/10.1021/nn5020787] [PMID: 24988275]

[54]   Godier-Furnémont AFMT, Martens TP, Koeckert MS, *et al.* Composite scaffold provides a cell delivery platform for cardiovascular repair. Proc Natl Acad Sci USA 2011; 108(19): 7974-9.
[http://dx.doi.org/10.1073/pnas.1104619108] [PMID: 21508321]

[55]   Singelyn JMSP, Sundaramurthy P, Johnson TD, *et al.* Catheter-deliverable hydrogel derived from decellularized ventricular extracellular matrix increases endogenous cardiomyocytes and preserves cardiac function post-myocardial infarction. J Am Coll Cardiol 2012; 59(8): 751-63.
[http://dx.doi.org/10.1016/j.jacc.2011.10.888] [PMID: 22340268]

[56]   Jia J, Richards DJ, Pollard S, *et al.* Engineering alginate as bioink for bioprinting. Acta Biomater 2014; 10(10): 4323-31.
[http://dx.doi.org/10.1016/j.actbio.2014.06.034] [PMID: 24998183]

[57]   Kraehenbuehl TPZP, Zammaretti P, Van der Vlies AJ, *et al.* Three-dimensional extracellular matrix-directed cardioprogenitor differentiation: systematic modulation of a synthetic cell-responsive PEG-hydrogel. Biomaterials 2008; 29(18): 2757-66.
[http://dx.doi.org/10.1016/j.biomaterials.2008.03.016] [PMID: 18396331]

[58]   Leor J, Tuvia S, Guetta V, *et al.* Intracoronary injection of *in situ* forming alginate hydrogel reverses left ventricular remodeling after myocardial infarction in Swine. J Am Coll Cardiol 2009; 54(11): 1014-23.
[http://dx.doi.org/10.1016/j.jacc.2009.06.010] [PMID: 19729119]

[59]   Mayfield AETE, Tilokee EL, Latham N, *et al.* The effect of encapsulation of cardiac stem cells within matrix-enriched hydrogel capsules on cell survival, post-ischemic cell retention and cardiac function. Biomaterials 2014; 35(1): 133-42.
[http://dx.doi.org/10.1016/j.biomaterials.2013.09.085] [PMID: 24099706]

[60]   Karoubi G, Ormiston ML, Stewart DJ, Courtman DW. Single-cell hydrogel encapsulation for enhanced survival of human marrow stromal cells. Biomaterials 2009; 30(29): 5445-55.
[http://dx.doi.org/10.1016/j.biomaterials.2009.06.035] [PMID: 19595454]

[61]   Cheng K, Li TS, Malliaras K, Davis DR, Zhang Y, Marbán E. Magnetic targeting enhances engraftment and functional benefit of iron-labeled cardiosphere-derived cells in myocardial infarction. Circ Res 2010; 106(10): 1570-81.
[http://dx.doi.org/10.1161/CIRCRESAHA.109.212589] [PMID: 20378859]

[62]   Yokoyama R, Ii M, Masuda M, *et al.* Cardiac Regeneration by Statin-Polymer Nanoparticle-Loaded Adipose-Derived Stem Cell Therapy in Myocardial Infarction. Stem Cells Transl Med 2019; 8(10): 1055-67.
[http://dx.doi.org/10.1002/sctm.18-0244] [PMID: 31157513]

[63]   Lee J-RPB-W, Park BW, Kim J, *et al.* Nanovesicles derived from iron oxide nanoparticles-incorporated mesenchymal stem cells for cardiac repair. Sci Adv 2020; 6(18): eaaz0952.
[http://dx.doi.org/10.1126/sciadv.aaz0952] [PMID: 32494669]

[64]   Vandergriff ACHT, Hensley TM, Henry ET, *et al.* Magnetic targeting of cardiosphere-derived stem cells with ferumoxytol nanoparticles for treating rats with myocardial infarction. Biomaterials 2014; 35(30): 8528-39.

[http://dx.doi.org/10.1016/j.biomaterials.2014.06.031] [PMID: 25043570]

[65] Dvir T, Timko BP, Brigham MD, *et al.* Nanowired three-dimensional cardiac patches. Nat Nanotechnol 2011; 6(11): 720-5.
[http://dx.doi.org/10.1038/nnano.2011.160] [PMID: 21946708]

[66] Feiner R, Engel L, Fleischer S, *et al.* Engineered hybrid cardiac patches with multifunctional electronics for online monitoring and regulation of tissue function. Nat Mater 2016; 15(6): 679-85.
[http://dx.doi.org/10.1038/nmat4590] [PMID: 26974408]

CHAPTER 13

Stem Cell Engineering Ability to Promote Cardiac Regenerative Activity

Ranjita Misra[1] and **Fahima Dilnawaz**[2,*]

[1] *Centre for Molecular and Nanomedical Sciences, Sathyabama Institute of Science and Technology, Chennai-600119, Tamil Nadu, India*

[2] *Laboratory of Nanomedicine, Institute of Life Sciences, Nalco Square, Chandrasekharpur, Bhubaneswar-751023, Odisha, India*

Abstract: The heart of adult humans is usually less capable of regeneration; several strategies have been used for the repairment of a damaged heart and to recover its function. However, stem cell technology showed a promising approach for cardiac therapy. More advanced strategies are used for improved stem cell-mediated cardiac regenerative therapy and to develop vascularization between scaffold (established by 3D engineered techniques) and host hearts. Through understanding the cellular and molecular mechanisms regulating heart regeneration, considerable progress has been made, which offers potentiality in controlling cardiac remodeling and redirecting the adult human heart towards a regenerative state.

Keywords: Cardiac regeneration, Cardiomyocytes, Mesenchymal stem cells, Pluripotent stem cells, Scaffold.

INTRODUCTION

The main reason behind heart failure is the irrecoverable damage to contractile heart muscles. To date, medicinal or surgical modalities are the only essentially available options for heart diseases [1]. In the year 1990, transplantation of syngeneic organism's cardiomyocytes (CMs) has shown to improve the function of the left ventricle in animal models of myocardial infarction [2]. Still, clinically there was no useful source of contractile cells. The maintenance of mammalian cardiomyocytes requires sophisticated routine protocols to keep alive for several days and always require the dissociation of neonatal rodent myocardium. Although isolation of adult CMs has been documented the cultivation of human CMs has been criticized a lot leading to futile research.

* **Corresponding author Fahima Dilnawaz:** Laboratory of Nanomedicine, Institute of Life Sciences, Nalco Square, Chandrasekharpur, Bhubaneswar 751023; Tel: +91-674 – 2304341; E-mail: fahimadilnawaz@gmail.com

Fahima Dilnawaz and Zeenat Iqbal (Eds.)

Mostly, the donor CMs are of allogeneic origin that raises the problem of immune rejection. Thus, the concept of using skeletal myoblasts for replacing CMs has become the topic of interest. However, the idea of using skeletal myoblasts failed because these cells are lacking with cardiomyocytes specific ion channels that are crucial for the electrical link with native CMs [3]. Till now, many investigations have reported the vast research on the derivation of CMs from numerous adult stem or progenitor cells [4, 5]. However, these are mainly disappointing at preclinical and clinical experiments. As compared to the presently used therapy, stem cell-based therapy has shown tremendous potential in enhancing and supporting the process of cardiac repair. Thus, stem cells afford the basis for complete regeneration of damaged cardiac tissue [6]. Although stem cells use in the context of cardiac tissue regeneration is highly appreciable. However, there exist many challenges and problems in cell-based therapy for CVDs. The analysis of current trials depicts that there exist a number of reasons behind the least success in cell-based therapy that includes patient's inconsistency *i.e.* variation in cell population choice, lower number isolation of cells and slow replicative potential. Moreover, the capacity of regeneration decreases with age, and also the delivery of enough numbers of the cell to the injury site is also a difficult task [7]. Thus, there is an urgent need for the improvement in the therapeutic properties of the used cell-based strategies in order to enhance the process of cardiac regeneration. To deal with the issue, stem cell engineering approaches provide solutions to overpower the present limitations. Particularly, the major goal of the engineering approaches has uniquely able to regulate the biochemical and biophysical characteristics of materials used in stem cell-based therapies [8]. Bioengineering strategies fill an exclusive environment for stem cell research by observing the dynamic behaviour of stem cell populations, which can be defined and manipulated strategically with the help of computational models in order to achieve desirable properties [9]. The eventual goal of stem cell bioengineering is to develop approaches to activate the populations of stem cells and allow probable control in regulating the fate of stem cells. This will set strategic engineering of the microenvironment for getting robust results using stem cell population for cardiac regeneration (Fig. **1**).

Moreover, bioengineering approaches can be useful to get a broad systems-level knowledge that is functional within the stem cells. It also helps in the understanding of rules that guide intracellular and cell-environment interactions that lead to the development of tissues and organs. Bioengineering strategies also help in improving stem cell survival and engraftment. The design of advanced materials can help in achieving the regulatory standards that increase the scale needed for commercialization. In this chapter, we will describe the role of stem cells in cardiac regeneration and how the stem cells are engineered for improving the stem cell-based therapies for cardiac tissue regeneration therapy.

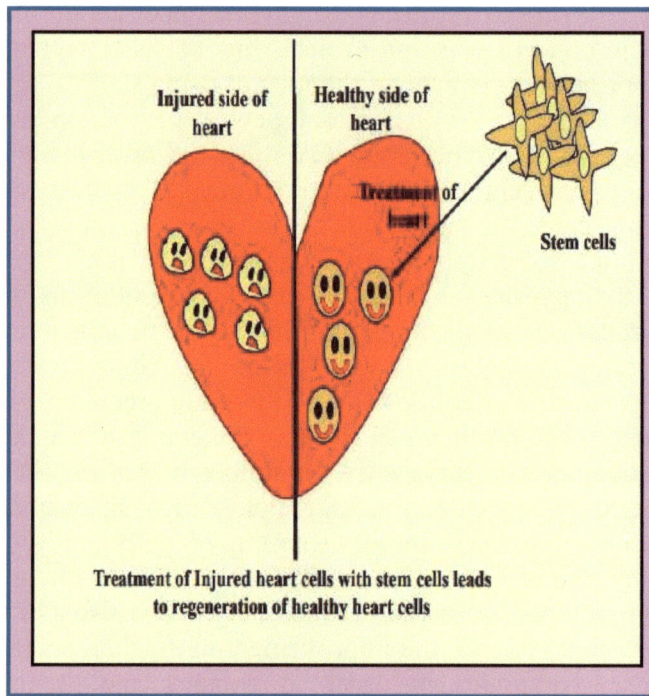

Fig. (1). Graphical illustration of stem cells based regeneration of injured heart.

STEM CELLS IN CARDIAC REGENERATIVE THERAPY

The therapeutic strategies for tissue regeneration have widely developed to combat the problem of damage or injury in different tissues or organs, which is caused due to any physical factors or the physiological ageing process in order to reduce the onset of its undesirable or negative effects. In this regard, stem cell based therapy has undoubtedly shown promising efficacy for the efficient management of a wide range of human diseases. Stem cells help in repair, replace or regeneration of damaged cells, tissues and organs that help in restoring its reduced function, which arises due to the effect of disease, ageing, trauma and defects [7]. Thus, stem cells have remained one of the major choices of clinicians and investigators for tissue regeneration therapy. Although many challenges exist in the clinical application of stem cell therapy, as evidenced from limited success obtained for human disease treatment till now [10]. The experimental and clinical study results are mainly challenged by a number of issues. Most significantly, a thorough understanding of stem cell biology has also shown the potential role of vesicular systems formed by stem cells such as exosomes and microvesicles. These vesicular systems are presently considered as a major form of wireless transformation of biological information between the microenvironment and the stem cells [11]. Regarding cardiac regenerative therapy, mainly two different groups of stem cells (SCs) are used, such as multipotent adult stem cells and pluripotent embryonic stem cells (ESCs) and induced pluripotent stem cells (iPSCs) [12]. In this case, either differentiated cells are used for transplantation, or the cells get differentiation after transplantation. Both the groups of cells have potential therapeutic properties with several advantages and disadvantages. ESCs and iPSCs have the advantage of having pluripotency, better *in vitro* expansion, easily available in high numbers and easy to create cell banks [13]. Moreover, iPSCs can be used for autologous transplantation. However, it may lead to the formation of teratoma due to the presence of remainders of iPSCs in the final or impaired differentiation cell fraction. Furthermore, it requires a prolonged time for culturing of these cells in order to get the final therapeutic product. This, in turn, leads to the production of miRNAs which are found in many cancers and becoming the reason for the development of genetic and epigenetic abnormalities. More significantly, the allogenic ESCs use raises the complication of immune reactions [14]. Additionally, it is provoking many legal and ethical debates for decades. In contrast, different stem and progenitor cells derived from several sources such as blood or solid tissues, bone marrow cells constitute the adult SC group. The most commonly used adult SCs are cardiac SCs (CSCs), bone marrow SCs, endothelial progenitor cells, mesenchymal stem cells and hematopoietic cells. The use of adult SCs for cardiac therapy has developed very effective and it is going to be in translation clinically very soon. A vast number of preclinical and clinical studies have developed many encouraging results with the use of adult SCs and progenitor cell transplantation in cardiac regeneration treatment.

THE NEED OF STEM CELL ENGINEERING FOR BETTER CARDIAC REGENERATION

Stem cell-based treatments have the tremendous potency to transform into medication that is capable of regeneration of patient-specific damaged tissues. That allows the cure of many intractable diseases such as diabetes, neurodegeneration disorders, and muscular dystrophies. The speedy progress in stem cell research from the last two decades has developed methods to use cells from mature cell types and even organs of the patients. This led to utilize the native regenerative capacity of the patient's own somatic stem cells found in their tissues. One more strategy, *i.e.*, the development of induced pluripotent stem (iPS) cells in which mature cells are taken from the skin or blood of patients, and then the cells are reprogrammed to an immature embryonic state [15]. These embryonic state cells can be able to differentiate into any kind of cells or adult tissues. Thus, the iPSC strategy provides a goal for the development of personalized medicine that can be used for the repairment of the damaged tissue or can be used as a diagnostic tool for screening of the drugs for deciding the treatment of patients made by the physicians.

Effective investigations on stem cell therapies translation to patients from last many years have raised the expectation that approaches for regenerative medicine can treat some most difficult diseases. Newly, genetically altered keratinocyte cultures comprising epidermal stem cells regenerated above 80% of the skin surface area of a patient with the lethal blistering disease. In other instances, embryonic stem (ES) cells or iPS cells isolated from patients have been transplanted into the eye that can differentiate into retinal pigment epithelial cells. Consequently, this enhanced the vision of patients who are in high danger of getting lost in visibility owing to macular degeneration. Regardless of such extremely revealed and stimulating studies of achievement, most of the clinical trials using stem cells till to date have not attained regulatory sanction and commercialization as stem cell therapies [16]. Though more than cents of clinical trials are listed with the US Food and Drug Administration (FDA), however, only umbilical cord blood-derived haematopoietic progenitors are FDA-approved stem cell products. This may be due to lengthy regulatory hurdles and also due to biological obstacles [17].

Although, considerable efforts have been achieved in stem cell biology. However, there remain many challenges that limit the potential clinical application of stem cell-based therapies. The hurdles that limit the translation of stem cell therapies to the clinic involve the maintenance of large number expansion of stem cells for transplantation, proper control of the state of the cells both before and after transplantation and safety of the cells during and post-delivery into the patients. The additional bottleneck is represented by the disappointment in replicating the regenerative properties by neural stem cells at the clinical level thus, showing the difficulties in the production and translation of stem cells for use in patients.

In order to overcome these current limitations engineering approaches, offer many solutions. Particularly, advancement in materials science has given solution in order to control the biochemical and biophysical properties of applied materials in stem cell-based therapies. The properties of the materials can easily be manipulated to form an artificial environment to grow naïve stem cells and also help in efficient differentiation of stem cells into required mature cell types. Stem cell therapy (SCT) is comprised of advanced therapy medicinal products (ATMPs), accompanied by gene therapy and tissue-engineered products [10]. ATMPs are an actual invention, being the exclusive chance for those ailments where medically effective treatments were missing.

The survivability and engraftment of stem cells can be improved with the use of biomaterials during transplantation. Moreover, the controlled properties of these biomaterials help in enhancing the regenerative capacity of the delivered stem cells [18]. Thus, for the success of stem cell therapy, many investigators are sicking the help of engineering approaches for achieving a potential solution. In this context, a tissue engineering tactic could be helpful through the whole procedure of development and regeneration of delivered therapeutic stem cells for the cardiac cells or tissues [19]. The biomaterials could not only help in delivering the stem cells, but also could provide support for the maturation of embryonic stem cells before the transplantation. There exist different approaches to engineer the heart tissue, such as seeding of stem cells in scaffolds, hydrogels, prefabricated synthetic matrices, *etc.*

ROLE OF NANOTECHNOLOGY IN STEM CELL ENGINEERING

Cardiac researchers and cardiologists are studying to implement various ideas of treating cardiomyopathies (heart muscle disease, in which it is harder for the heart to pump blood to the rest of the body) by developing cardiomyocytes (CMs) that are able to proliferate and form new contractile force [20]. The mammalian heart's regenerative potential is a type of process that depends on age which is also inadequate in new-borns [21]. Further insufficiency of the heart muscle's capacity to function in return in injured case [22]. Additionally, the regenerative potential of cardiac muscle remains unclear because of the appropriate understanding of the resident progenitor cell's biology [23]. Recently stem cells have developed as a foremost treatment choice and are engaged in the application of regenerative medicine as because of the self-renewal and proliferation capability as well as having the ability to develop into multiple cell types to establish viable tissue. Restricted proliferation and self-healing ability of cardiomyocytes contribute less to the injuries of the heart which are often permanent. In this regard stem cell-based cardiovascular therapy has become quite important. Commonly derived stem cells are from bone marrow cells, inducible pluripotent stem cells, resident cardiac stem cells, mesenchymal or adipose tissue-derived stem cells, skeletal myoblasts, and circulating stem cells that can be injected directly to the site of CVD. Human induced pluripotent stem cells (hiPSCs) are mainly delivered by cell injections for various applications [24, 25], cell patches [26], cell sheets [27] and cell-matrix inoculation [28]. Due to the deficiency of strong pre-clinical mechanism studies, there is disappointment in cardiac treatment [29]. Conventional stem cell therapies are mostly linked with major side effects owing to the inherent noxious effect of the drugs, their wide range of action and uncontrolled delivery [30]. Current tissue engineering methods face many obstacles because of inappropriate biomaterials leading to ineffective cell growth, which in turn could not achieve proper physiological architectures and remains unstable due to lacking in growth factors secretion that helps in cell contact and appropriate response [31]. Nanotechnology-based therapeutic application are the leading entities due to their characteristic size-dependent properties as well as unique physico-chemical characteristics. It has shown enormous promise for the diagnosis and therapy of cardiovascular disease (CVDs). In this context designing of the nanoparticles which can target contractile component of the heart and offers suitable solutions to overcome the limitation of the current therapies. With the advent of nanoparticle-based therapy, various custom made nano-constructs have been used for various applications in medical field, in turn giving the opportunity for carrying and delivering several kinds of cargos. Nanotechnological application in the field of regenerative tissue engineering particularly deals with enhancement of heart's biological, electrical and mechanical properties as well as gene delivery [32].

STEM CELLS LABELLING

Two different types of stem cells (SCs) are presently used for cardiac regenerative medicine: (i) multipotent adult SCs and (ii) pluripotent embryonic SCs (ESCs) and induced pluripotent SCs (iPSCs), and differentiated derivatives are being explored for transplantation [29, 33]. Both the above categories have some potential merits and demerits [33]. Stem cell labelling is done by magnetically targeted delivery, wherein infers loading of SCs with magnetic responsive particles to facilitate the guidance of cells at the target area [34]. Various research groups have attempted successful demonstration of stem cell targeting. For acute or chronic ischemic cardiomyopathy, transplantation of SC is a promising therapeutic strategy; however, it has limitations due to low retention and engraftment efficiency as well as substantial initial "wash-out" of cells from coronary blood flow and heart contraction. Therefore, in order to increase the retaining and engraftment, the labelling of human cardiosphere-derived stem cells (hCDCs) was done by using FDA-approved ferumoxytol nanoparticles Feraheme(®) (F) in heparin (H) and protamine (P) presence. Vandergriff and coworkers demonstrated that with magnetic targeting, cell SC retention has increased at the infarcted rat myocardium ~ 4-fold compared to control, where no magnet was applied [35]. In another approach Cheng *et al.* demonstrated successful intracoronary (IC) delivery and retention of cells by targeting with a magnetic system, for which rat cardiosphere-derived cells labelled with iron microspheres and were injected into the left ventricular cavity of syngeneic rats during brief aortic clamping. Application of external magnet above the heart during the procedure elevated the cell retention ~ 6 fold without the elevation of serum troponin I levels [36]. To know the optimum intensity of the magnetic targeting, Shen *et al.* investigated the effects of intensities of magnetic targeting for mesenchymal stem cell (MSC) on cell transplantation using changed magnetic intensities. The study revealed that retention of cells was enhanced by magnetic targeting in a magnetic field strength-dependent manner. Microembolization and consequent weakening of the functional profits of cell transplantation take place with too high magnetic intensity [37]. Another significant study targeted nanomedicine strategy was applied by using superparamagnetic iron nanoparticles which are conjugated with two different kinds of antibodies, one is CD45+ therapeutic endogenous SCs that is against antigens on therapeutic cells and other is directed towards injured cells of cardiomyocytes in order to develop magnetic bifunctional cell engager (MagBICE). They observed ~10-fold increase in targeting of CD45+ cells to the region of infraction and also an enhancement in the therapeutic activity with the intravenous injection of the particles along with the application of magnetic field to the site of myocardial infarction in rats. These antibodies get linked the injured cells, while the core of iron MagBICE allows physical enrichment and imaging, and magnetic targeting enhanced it further leads to increased benefits functionally. Thus MagBICE represents a generalizable platform technology for regenerative medicine [36]. It is indispensable for tracking the fate of injected cells with different imaging methods for the assessment of the distribution of stem cells in cardiac therapy. Labeling of stem cells is mostly studied by employing contrast agents of superparamagnetic iron oxide nanoparticles (SPIONs) [38]. Bone marrow mesenchymal stem cells (BMSCs) labelled with SPIO were used in MRI to track myocardial infarction for different time courses in a rat model. They documented that the signal strength was declined with time while the signal area gradually extended into the infarcted myocardium [39]. Numerous *in vitro* and preclinical studies magnetic nanoparticles are used; the study revealed that augmented concentrations of iron can rise the free radicals level intracellularly in a dose-dependent manner [40]. Although application of strong magnetic fields can have augmenting or hindering effects on biological systems or which can direct it towards the formation of toxic masses from intracellularly located magnetic particles [40, 41]. In this process there are certain limitation for using magnetic nanoparticles for imaging transplanted SCs, at certain point of time, it is difficult to distinguish magnetized viable and dead cells; because long-term MRI-based follow-up of injected cells is compromised due to the leakage of iron particles or their uptake by macrophages [42 - 44]. To overcome this problem, customization of MR reporter genes might be helpful. Overexpression of the transferrin receptor or ferritin, which is a marker is generally used to enhance the intracellular concentration of iron which intensely augment contrast in MRI tracking [45, 46].

ULTRASOUND-BASED DELIVERY OF STEM CELLS

Cell targeting by using the ultrasound method is considered as a novel technique to mostly increasing the cell retention and engraftment at the injury site. In this process, gas-filled microbubbles are involved in the SCs, which become very susceptible to acoustic radiation forces. With the help of ultrasound catheter intracoronary injection, the SCs can be positioned and detained at the site of injury [47, 48]. A study conducted by Tong *et al.*, showed that, the combination of ultrasound with nitric oxide (NO) micro-bubble destruction could be applied for cell transplantation, which can proficiently help the MSC homing into the infarcted myocardium [48]. Restoration of functional endothelium is an essential condition for avoiding delayed stent thrombosis. Tome *et al*. developed an innovative technique of ultrasound-generated acoustic radiation force for targeted delivery of stem cells at the arterial injury site. In which the surface of MSCs was coated with cationic gas-filled lipid microbubbles (mb-MSC) by electrostatic interaction and with the aid of ultrasound are applied in a rabbit model. There was 150-fold enrichment of cells at the endoluminal surface, whereas no effect was observed on mb-MSCs in the absence of ultrasound [47]. In another study, noteworthy enhancement of cardiac functions and cardiac remodeling after MI in dog was observed with enhanced efficiency of cell delivery and increased MSC engraftment *via* microbubble/ultrasound system [49]. Targeted delivery was done with designed antibody coated microbubbles, which can target both the SC-specific marker CD90 and an adhesion molecule expressed on endothelial cells within the infarcted area. This active targeting system permits precise delivery to the injured myocardium in a rat MI model, whereas nearly no cells were present in the non-infarcted area [50].

SCAFFOLDS FOR STEM CELLS DELIVERY

A biological scaffold means a three-dimensional structure that provides support. These scaffolds can mimic the structural, chemical, and physical environment in which cells that are formed can be used either to repair or replace the native tissues. In the case of cardiac tissue scaffold or dynamic development of cardiomyocytes, various factors are responsible such as characteristics of extracellular matrix, shape, growth hormones, physical stresses like cell-cell tension and electrical stimulation are significant [51]. *In vitro* cell grafts are prepared with no additional factors, which are less effective for acute or chronic cardiac dysfunction treatment *in vivo*. Nanotechnology-mediated scaffold preparation has been done by various research groups that can help their differentiation into functional myocardium. Recent advances in nanofabrication techniques enable the design and fabrication of scaffolding materials that have similar structural and mechanical properties as ECM environment in *in vivo*. Hydrogels are formed from the network of polymer hydrophilic chains held together by cross-linking. The 3D polymeric network of hydrogel undergoes swelling with the addition of water into it. The hydrogel can be of different types like gelatin, alginate, collagen, fibrin, and so forth [52]. Kim *et al*. developed anisotropically nanofabricated substratum (ANFS) biocompatible polyethylene glycol (PEG) hydrogel arrays that imitate the physiological characteristics of native myocardial tissue ECM [51]. Chen *et al*. utilized bone marrow-derived MSCs (BM-MSCs) with hydrogel composite biomaterial injection into infarcted myocardium for the improvement of cardiac functioning by preventing left ventricular (LV) remodelling [53]. Santhakumar *et al*. used cardiogel, a cardiac fibroblast-derived extracellular matrix (ECM) that helps in cardiomyogenic differentiation, angiogenesis of BMSCs, which offer safety against oxidative stress and preserved the structure of the matrix by yielding greater amounts of collagen and protein [54]. Jeffords *et al*. utilized cardiac matrix hydrogel as an injectable biomaterial as it possesses cardiac-specific extracellular matrix composition and it facilitates neovascularization for the improvement of cardiac repair. For enhancement of endothelial differentiation of stem cells, a natural compound genipin is being crosslinked for the mechanical properties of the cardiac hydrogel. The culture of human mesenchymal stem cells (hMSCs) showed high viability, and promotes quick vascularization for cardiac infarction treatment [55]. Bai *et al*. studied the effect of temperature-sensitive ECM hydrogels using decellularized heart matrix, enhanced the fate of cardiomyogenic cells toward benefiting myocardial repair by augmenting stem cell therapy [56]. Encapsulation of stem cell in hydrogels has recently received great attention for minimally invasive administration for enhancement of therapeutic efficacy. Mayfield *et al*., encapsulated cardiac stem cells within matrix-enriched hydrogel capsules for post-ischemic cell retention and cardiac function. Encapsulated CSCs have shown more secretion of cardio-protective and pro-angiogenic cytokines. Thus, encapsulation of CSC have been reported boosting the acute engraftment with a long-term survivability after injection in a myocardial infracted *in vivo* model [57]. Nanofibers are formulated from various polymers and hence have distinct physical characteristics and application capacities. The size of nanofibre is crucial because it can impact on the process of cell differentiation. Hosseinkhani *et al*., grew mesenchymal stem cells on nanofibers and those were grown profusely on nanofibers that led to favored differentiation of stem cells into chondrocytes, signifying the outcome of extracellular structure for controlling differentiation [58]. The structure and design of the nanoscale scaffold also impact the cell maturation [59]. In small and large animals, biodegradable scaffolds like matrigel, cardiogel, fibrin, or collagen support adhesion, differentiation, and proliferation of various types of stem cells, including ESCs and bone marrow-derived SCs [60]. With adipose-derived MSCs, co-injection with fibrin augmented the retention of cells significantly with four weeks of transplantation into murine hearts [61]. Simpson *et al*., demonstrated that human mesenchymal stem cells (hMSCs) in a collagen matrix, when applied to the heart, performed better than the same cells grown in monolayer condition and then injected directly for cardiac cell replacement in a myocardial infarcted rat model. The culture of hMSC in collagen patches also enhanced the angiogenic response. Transplantation of hMSC patches to the infarcted heart of rat, illustrated better-left ventricle (LV) remodelling and function [62]. Exosomes are cell-derived vesicles that are actively involved for signal transduction, immune responses, antigen presentation, and would healing among other cellular physiological processes such as, transport proteins, lipids, DNA, and RNA *etc* has the potential capacity for bioactive therapies [63]. To improve cardiac function after MI recently, exosomes derived from stem cells when introduced into scaffolds contribute as regulator of cardiac remodelling to establish circulatory scaffolds [64]. Looking at the wide range of cellular activity hucMSC-derived exosomes have been shown to exert cardioprotective effects [65]. Thermosensitive injectable hydrogel are based on *N*-acryloxysuccinimide, *N*-isopropylacrylamide, poly(trimethylene carbonate)-hydroxyethyl methacrylate and acrylic acid are used for delivering MSCs into the heart, where it can be differentiated into cardiac cells with high efficacy [66].

FUTURE DIRECTIONS

The finding of numerous resident stem cell populations and their therapeutic skill has generated a wealth of research scope towards the potentiality of regenerating injured cardiac tissue. For attenuating remodeling and transforming inert scar into biochemically functional myocardium, stem cell therapy has revealed great promise. The translational potential of stem cell therapy into clinical application is not an easy task, and it requires various obstacles to overpower before this treatment reaches its full potential. For true regeneration, a considerable percentage of the stem cells are required which can remain functionally viable to be differentiated. With current treatment modality in conjunction with stem cell therapy may help to enhance the quality of life in CVD patients. Although much more work needs to be done.

CONCLUSION

The heart is an extremely complex organ, and its related disease is also highly complex, and the technique influencing its regeneration depends mainly on many variables. Stem cell-based regeneration has shown immense potential for cardiac disease. Nano-enabled approaches (*e.g.*, nanomaterials, nano-featured surfaces) immensely contribute to developing appropriate scaffolding biomaterials which can regulate stem cells' microenvironment for achieving functional therapeutic outcomes. Research studies have demonstrated fruitful therapeutic promising application with integration of advanced biomaterials and stem cells for regeneration of damaged myocardium. Further, by using induced pluripotent stem cells, human cardiomyocytes are easy to generate in mass, which is an immensely capable approach for three-dimensional heart regeneration. Using this technique cardiomyocytes can be effectively engrafted onto the cardiac scaffolds. Complete myocardial regeneration in order to obtain an acellular human heart matrix is still in its infancy, and thus, it requires more studies before this system can be translated clinically in the near future.

CONSENT FOR PUBLICATION

Not Applicable.

CONFLICT OF INTEREST

The author confirms that this chapter contents have no conflict of interest.

ACKNOWLEDGEMENT

FD gratefully acknowledges the Dept. of Science and Technology, Govt. of India, for the financial grant [SR/WOS-A/LS-448/2017(G)] in the form of a women scientist fellowship (WOS-A).

REFERENCES

[1]   Isomi M, Sadahiro T, Ieda M. Progress and challenge of cardiac regeneration to treat heart failure. J Cardiol 2019; 73(2): 97-101.
[http://dx.doi.org/10.1016/j.jjcc.2018.10.002] [PMID: 30420106]

[2]   Lösse B. Indications and selection criteria for cardiac transplantation. Thorac Cardiovasc Surg 1990; 38(5): 276-9.
[http://dx.doi.org/10.1055/s-2007-1014034] [PMID: 2264035]

[3]   Fu J-D, Srivastava D. Direct reprogramming of fibroblasts into cardiomyocytes for cardiac regenerative medicine. Circ J 2015; 79(2): 245-54.
[http://dx.doi.org/10.1253/circj.CJ-14-1372] [PMID: 25744738]

[4]   Mills RJ, Titmarsh DM, Koenig X, *et al.* Functional screening in human cardiac organoids reveals a metabolic mechanism for cardiomyocyte cell cycle arrest. Proc Natl Acad Sci USA 2017; 114(40): E8372-81.
[http://dx.doi.org/10.1073/pnas.1707316114] [PMID: 28916735]

[5]   Miyawaki A, Obana M, Mitsuhara Y, *et al.* Adult murine cardiomyocytes exhibit regenerative activity with cell cycle reentry through STAT3 in the healing process of myocarditis. Sci Rep 2017; 7(1): 1407.
[http://dx.doi.org/10.1038/s41598-017-01426-8] [PMID: 28469272]

[6]   Jeffords ME, Wu J, Shah M, Hong Y, Zhang G. Tailoring material properties of cardiac matrix hydrogels to induce endothelial differentiation of human mesenchymal stem cells. ACS Appl Mater Interfaces 2015; 7(20): 11053-61.
[http://dx.doi.org/10.1021/acsami.5b03195] [PMID: 25946697]

[7]   Carvalho E, Verma P, Hourigan K, Banerjee R. Myocardial infarction: stem cell transplantation for cardiac regeneration. Regen Med 2015; 10(8): 1025-43.
[http://dx.doi.org/10.2217/rme.15.63] [PMID: 26563414]

[8]   Qasim M, Haq F, Kang MH, Kim JH. 3D printing approaches for cardiac tissue engineering and role of immune modulation in tissue regeneration. Int J Nanomedicine 2019; 14: 1311-33.
[http://dx.doi.org/10.2147/IJN.S189587] [PMID: 30863063]

[9]   Guyette JP, Charest JM, Mills RW, *et al.* Bioengineering Human Myocardium on Native Extracellular Matrix. Circ Res 2016; 118(1): 56-72.
[http://dx.doi.org/10.1161/CIRCRESAHA.115.306874] [PMID: 26503464]

[10] Weinberger F, Mannhardt I, Eschenhagen T. Engineering Cardiac Muscle Tissue: A Maturating Field of Research. Circ Res 2017; 120(9): 1487-500.
[http://dx.doi.org/10.1161/CIRCRESAHA.117.310738] [PMID: 28450366]

[11] Tang J, Shen D, Caranasos TG, *et al.* Therapeutic microparticles functionalized with biomimetic cardiac stem cell membranes and secretome. Nat Commun 2017; 8: 13724.
[http://dx.doi.org/10.1038/ncomms13724] [PMID: 28045024]

[12] Ishigami M, Masumoto H, Ikuno T, *et al.* Human iPS cell-derived cardiac tissue sheets for functional restoration of infarcted porcine hearts. PLoS One 2018; 13(8): e0201650.
[http://dx.doi.org/10.1371/journal.pone.0201650] [PMID: 30071102]

[13] Duran AG, Reidell O, Stachelscheid H, *et al.* Regenerative Medicine/Cardiac Cell Therapy: Pluripotent Stem Cells. Thorac Cardiovasc Surg 2018; 66(1): 53-62.
[http://dx.doi.org/10.1055/s-0037-1608761] [PMID: 29216651]

[14] Bargehr J, Ong LP, Colzani M, *et al.* Epicardial cells derived from human embryonic stem cells augment cardiomyocyte-driven heart regeneration. Nat Biotechnol 2019; 37(8): 895-906.
[http://dx.doi.org/10.1038/s41587-019-0197-9] [PMID: 31375810]

[15] Shiba Y, Gomibuchi T, Seto T, *et al.* Allogeneic transplantation of iPS cell-derived cardiomyocytes regenerates primate hearts. Nature 2016; 538(7625): 388-91.
[http://dx.doi.org/10.1038/nature19815] [PMID: 27723741]

[16] https://clinicaltrials.gov

[17] Bagno L, Hatzistergos KE, Balkan W, Hare JM. Mesenchymal Stem Cell-Based Therapy for Cardiovascular Disease: Progress and Challenges. Mol Ther 2018; 26(7): 1610-23.
[http://dx.doi.org/10.1016/j.ymthe.2018.05.009] [PMID: 29807782]

[18] Kharaziha M, Memic A, Akbari M, Brafman DA, Nikkhah M. Nano-Enabled Approaches for Stem Cell-Based Cardiac Tissue Engineering. Adv Healthc Mater 2016; 5(13): 1533-53.
[http://dx.doi.org/10.1002/adhm.201600088] [PMID: 27199266]

[19] Bai R, Tian L, Li Y, *et al.* Combining ECM Hydrogels of Cardiac Bioactivity with Stem Cells of High Cardiomyogenic Potential for Myocardial Repair. Stem Cells Int 2019; 2019: 6708435.
[http://dx.doi.org/10.1155/2019/6708435] [PMID: 31772589]

[20] Hashmi S, Ahmad HR. Molecular switch model for cardiomyocyte proliferation. Cell Regen (Lond) 2019; 8(1): 12-20.
[http://dx.doi.org/10.1016/j.cr.2018.11.002] [PMID: 31205684]

[21] Porrello ER, Mahmoud AI, Simpson E, *et al.* Regulation of neonatal and adult mammalian heart regeneration by the miR-15 family. Proc Natl Acad Sci USA 2013; 110(1): 187-92.
[http://dx.doi.org/10.1073/pnas.1208863110] [PMID: 23248315]

[22] Eschenhagen T, Bolli R, Braun T, *et al.* Cardiomyocyte regeneration. Circulation 2017; 136(7): 680-6.
[http://dx.doi.org/10.1161/CIRCULATIONAHA.117.029343] [PMID: 28684531]

[23] Tzahor E, Poss KD. Cardiac regeneration strategies: Staying young at heart. Science 2017; 356(6342): 1035-9.
[http://dx.doi.org/10.1126/science.aam5894] [PMID: 28596337]

[24] Bartunek J, Terzic A, Davison BA, *et al.* CHART Program. Cardiopoietic cell therapy for advanced ischaemic heart failure: results at 39 weeks of the prospective, randomized, double blind, sham-controlled CHART-1 clinical trial. Eur Heart J 2017; 38(9): 648-60.
[PMID: 28025189]

[25] Butler J, Epstein SE, Greene SJ, *et al.* Intravenous allogeneic mesenchymal stem cells for nonischemic cardiomyopathy safety and efficacy results of a phase II-A randomized trial. Circ Res 2017; 120(2): 332-40.
[http://dx.doi.org/10.1161/CIRCRESAHA.116.309717] [PMID: 27856497]

[26]   Dolan EB, Hofmann B, de Vaal MH, *et al.* A bioresorbable biomaterial carrier and passive stabilization device to improve heart function post-myocardial infarction. Mater Sci Eng C 2019; 103: 109751.
       [http://dx.doi.org/10.1016/j.msec.2019.109751] [PMID: 31349422]

[27]   Miyagawa S, Domae K, Yoshikawa Y, *et al.* Phase I clinical trial of autologous stem cell-sheet transplantation therapy for treating cardiomyopathy. J Am Heart Assoc 2017; 6(4): e003918.
       [http://dx.doi.org/10.1161/JAHA.116.003918] [PMID: 28381469]

[28]   Traverse JH, Henry TD, Dib N, *et al.* First-in-man study of a cardiac extracellular matrix hydrogel in early and late myocardial infarction patients. JACC Basic Transl Sci 2019; 4(6): 659-69.
       [http://dx.doi.org/10.1016/j.jacbts.2019.07.012] [PMID: 31709316]

[29]   Menasché P, Vanneaux V, Hagège A, *et al.* Human embryonic stem cell-derived cardiac progenitors for severe heart failure treatment: first clinical case report. Eur Heart J 2015; 36(30): 2011-7.
       [http://dx.doi.org/10.1093/eurheartj/ehv189] [PMID: 25990469]

[30]   Jabir NRTS, Tabrez S, Ashraf GM, Shakil S, Damanhouri GA, Kamal MA. Nanotechnology-based approaches in anticancer research. Int J Nanomedicine 2012; 7: 4391-408.
       [PMID: 22927757]

[31]   Ikada Y. Challenges in tissue engineering. J R Soc Interface 2006; 3(10): 589-601.
       [http://dx.doi.org/10.1098/rsif.2006.0124] [PMID: 16971328]

[32]   Cassani M, Fernandes S, Vrbsky J, Ergir E, Cavalieri F, Forte G. Combining Nanomaterials and Developmental Pathways to Design New Treatments for Cardiac Regeneration: The Pulsing Heart of Advanced Therapies. Front Bioeng Biotechnol 2020; 8(323): 323.
       [http://dx.doi.org/10.3389/fbioe.2020.00323] [PMID: 32391340]

[33]   Lalit PA, Hei DJ, Raval AN, Kamp TJ. Induced pluripotent stem cells for post-myocardial infarction repair: remarkable opportunities and challenges. Circ Res 2014; 114(8): 1328-45.
       [http://dx.doi.org/10.1161/CIRCRESAHA.114.300556] [PMID: 24723658]

[34]   Lemcke H, Voronina N, Steinhoff G, David R. Recent Progress in Stem Cell Modification for Cardiac Regeneration. Stem Cells Int 2018; 2018: 1909346.
       [http://dx.doi.org/10.1155/2018/1909346] [PMID: 29535769]

[35]   Vandergriff AC, Hensley TM, Henry ET, *et al.* Magnetic targeting of cardiosphere-derived stem cells with ferumoxytol nanoparticles for treating rats with myocardial infarction. Biomaterials 2014; 35(30): 8528-39.
       [http://dx.doi.org/10.1016/j.biomaterials.2014.06.031] [PMID: 25043570]

[36]   Cheng K, Malliaras K, Li T-S, *et al.* Magnetic enhancement of cell retention, engraftment, and functional benefit after intracoronary delivery of cardiac-derived stem cells in a rat model of ischemia/reperfusion. Cell Transplant 2012; 21(6): 1121-35.
       [http://dx.doi.org/10.3727/096368911X627381] [PMID: 22405128]

[37]   Shen Y, Liu X, Huang Z, *et al.* Comparison of magnetic intensities for mesenchymal stem cell targeting therapy on ischemic myocardial repair: high magnetic intensity improves cell retention but has no additional functional benefit. Cell Transplant 2015; 24(10): 1981-97.
       [http://dx.doi.org/10.3727/096368914X685302] [PMID: 25375750]

[38]   Laurent S, Dutz S, Häfeli UO, Mahmoudi M. Magnetic fluid hyperthermia: focus on superparamagnetic iron oxide nanoparticles. Adv Colloid Interface Sci 2011; 166(1-2): 8-23.
       [http://dx.doi.org/10.1016/j.cis.2011.04.003] [PMID: 21601820]

[39]   Hua P, Wang Y-Y, Liu L-B, *et al.* In vivo magnetic resonance imaging tracking of transplanted superparamagnetic iron oxide-labeled bone marrow mesenchymal stem cells in rats with myocardial infarction. Mol Med Rep 2015; 11(1): 113-20.
       [http://dx.doi.org/10.3892/mmr.2014.2649] [PMID: 25323652]

[40]   Silva LHA, Cruz FF, Morales MM, Weiss DJ, Rocco PRM. Magnetic targeting as a strategy to

enhance therapeutic effects of mesenchymal stromal cells. Stem Cell Res Ther 2017; 8(1): 58.
[http://dx.doi.org/10.1186/s13287-017-0523-4] [PMID: 28279201]

[41]   Albuquerque WW, Costa RM, Fernandes TdeS, Porto AL. Evidences of the static magnetic field influence on cellular systems. Prog Biophys Mol Biol 2016; 121(1): 16-28.
[http://dx.doi.org/10.1016/j.pbiomolbio.2016.03.003] [PMID: 26975790]

[42]   Han C, Zhou J, Liang C, *et al.* Human umbilical cord mesenchymal stem cell derived exosomes encapsulated in functional peptide hydrogels promote cardiac repair. Biomater Sci 2019; 7(7): 2920-33.
[http://dx.doi.org/10.1039/C9BM00101H] [PMID: 31090763]

[43]   Kim D-H, Lipke EA, Kim P, *et al.* Nanoscale cues regulate the structure and function of macroscopic cardiac tissue constructs. Proc Natl Acad Sci USA 2010; 107(2): 565-70.
[http://dx.doi.org/10.1073/pnas.0906504107] [PMID: 20018748]

[44]   Naumova AV, Balu N, Yarnykh VL, Reinecke H, Murry CE, Yuan C. Magnetic resonance imaging tracking of graft survival in the infarcted heart: iron oxide particles *versus* ferritin overexpression approach. J Cardiovasc Pharmacol Ther 2014; 19(4): 358-67.
[http://dx.doi.org/10.1177/1074248414525999] [PMID: 24685664]

[45]   Santoso MR, Yang PC. Magnetic nanoparticles for targeting and imaging of stem cells in myocardial infarction. Stem Cells Int 2016; 2016: 4198790.
[http://dx.doi.org/10.1155/2016/4198790] [PMID: 27127519]

[46]   Cho IK, Wang S, Mao H, Chan AW. Genetic engineered molecular imaging probes for applications in cell therapy: emphasis on MRI approach. Am J Nucl Med Mol Imaging 2016; 6(5): 234-61.
[PMID: 27766183]

[47]   Lee CW, Choi SII, Lee SJ, *et al.* The effectiveness of ferritin as a contrast agent for celltracking MRI in mouse cancer models. Yonsei Med J 2017; 58(1): 51-8.
[http://dx.doi.org/10.3349/ymj.2017.58.1.51] [PMID: 27873495]

[48]   Toma C, Fisher A, Wang J, *et al.* Vascular endoluminal delivery of mesenchymal stem cells using acoustic radiation force. Tissue Eng Part A 2011; 17(9-10): 1457-64.
[http://dx.doi.org/10.1089/ten.tea.2010.0539] [PMID: 21247343]

[49]   Tong J, Ding J, Shen X, *et al.* Mesenchymal stem cell transplantation enhancement in myocardial infarction rat model under ultrasound combined with nitric oxide microbubbles. PLoS One 2013; 8(11): e80186.
[http://dx.doi.org/10.1371/journal.pone.0080186] [PMID: 24244646]

[50]   Chang X, Liu J, Liao X, Liu G. Ultrasound-mediated microbubble destruction enhances the therapeutic effect of intracoronary transplantation of bone marrow stem cells on myocardial infarction. Int J Clin Exp Pathol 2015; 8(2): 2221-34.
[PMID: 25973133]

[51]   Woudstra L, Krijnen PAJ, Bogaards SJP, *et al.* Development of a new therapeutic technique to direct stem cells to the infarcted heart using targeted microbubbles: StemBells. Stem Cell Res (Amst) 2016; 17(1): 6-15.
[http://dx.doi.org/10.1016/j.scr.2016.04.018] [PMID: 27186654]

[52]   Radhakrishnan J, Krishnan UM, Sethuraman S. Hydrogel based injectable scaffolds for cardiac tissue regeneration. Biotechnol Adv 2014; 32(2): 449-61.
[http://dx.doi.org/10.1016/j.biotechadv.2013.12.010] [PMID: 24406815]

[53]   Chen J, Guo R, Zhou Q, Wang T. Injection of composite with bone marrow-derived mesenchymal stem cells and a novel synthetic hydrogel after myocardial infarction: a protective role in left ventricle function. Kaohsiung J Med Sci 2014; 30(4): 173-80.
[http://dx.doi.org/10.1016/j.kjms.2013.12.004] [PMID: 24656157]

[54]   Santhakumar R, Vidyasekar P, Verma RS. Cardiogel: a nano-matrix scaffold with potential application

in cardiac regeneration using mesenchymal stem cells. PLoS One 2014; 9(12): e114697.
[http://dx.doi.org/10.1371/journal.pone.0114697] [PMID: 25521816]

[55]   Mayfield AE, Tilokee EL, Latham N, *et al.* The effect of encapsulation of cardiac stem cells within matrix-enriched hydrogel capsules on cell survival, post-ischemic cell retention and cardiac function. Biomaterials 2014; 35(1): 133-42.
[http://dx.doi.org/10.1016/j.biomaterials.2013.09.085] [PMID: 24099706]

[56]   Hosseinkhani H, Hosseinkhani M, Kobayashi H. Proliferation and differentiation of mesenchymal stem cells using self-assembled peptide amphiphile nanofibers. Biomed Mater 2006; 1(1): 8-15.
[http://dx.doi.org/10.1088/1748-6041/1/1/002] [PMID: 18458380]

[57]   Kim D-H, Kim P, Song I, *et al.* Guided three-dimensional growth of functional cardiomyocytes on polyethylene glycol nanostructures. Langmuir 2006; 22(12): 5419-26.
[http://dx.doi.org/10.1021/la060283u] [PMID: 16732672]

[58]   Fakoya AO, Fakoya J. New delivery systems of stem cells for vascular regeneration in ischemia. Front Cardiovasc Med 2017; 4: 7.
[http://dx.doi.org/10.3389/fcvm.2017.00007] [PMID: 28286751]

[59]   Zhang X, Wang H, Ma X, *et al.* Preservation of the cardiac function in infarcted rat hearts by the transplantation of adipose-derived stem cells with injectable fibrin scaffolds. Exp Biol Med (Maywood) 2010; 235(12): 1505-15.
[http://dx.doi.org/10.1258/ebm.2010.010175] [PMID: 21127347]

[60]   Simpson DL, Dudley SC Jr. Modulation of human mesenchymal stem cell function in a three-dimensional matrix promotes attenuation of adverse remodelling after myocardial infarction. J Tissue Eng Regen Med 2013; 7(3): 192-202.
[http://dx.doi.org/10.1002/term.511] [PMID: 22095744]

[61]   Théry C, Ostrowski M, Segura E. Membrane vesicles as conveyors of immune responses. Nat Rev Immunol 2009; 9(8): 581-93.
[http://dx.doi.org/10.1038/nri2567] [PMID: 19498381]

[62]   Jung JH, Fu X, Yang PC. Exosomes Generated From iPSC-Derivatives: New Direction for Stem Cell Therapy in Human Heart Diseases. Circ Res 2017; 120(2): 407-17.
[http://dx.doi.org/10.1161/CIRCRESAHA.116.309307] [PMID: 28104773]

[63]   Wang X-L, Zhao Y-Y, Sun L, *et al.* Exosomes derived from human umbilical cord mesenchymal stem cells improve myocardial repair *via* upregulation of Smad7. Int J Mol Med 2018; 41(5): 3063-72.
[http://dx.doi.org/10.3892/ijmm.2018.3496] [PMID: 29484378]

[64]   Li Z, Guo X, Palmer AF, Das H, Guan J. High-efficiency matrix modulus-induced cardiac differentiation of human mesenchymal stem cells inside a thermosensitive hydrogel. Acta Biomater 2012; 8(10): 3586-95.
[http://dx.doi.org/10.1016/j.actbio.2012.06.024] [PMID: 22729021]

[65]   Wang XL, Zhao YY, Sun L, *et al.* Exosomes derived from human umbilical cord mesenchymal stem cells improve myocardial repair *via* upregulation of Smad7. Int J Mol Med 2018; 41(5): 3063-72.
[http://dx.doi.org/10.3892/ijmm.2018.3496] [PMID: 29484378]

[66]   Li Z, Guo X, Palmer AF, Das H, Guan J. G.X. Li Z. High-efficiency matrix modulus-induced cardiac differentiation of human mesenchymal stem cells inside a thermosensitive hydrogel. Acta Biomater 2012; 8(10): 3586-95.
[http://dx.doi.org/10.1016/j.actbio.2012.06.024] [PMID: 22729021]

SUBJECT INDEX

A

Autonomy 70,72

B

Beneficence 70
Bioavailability 1, 2, 11, 20, 22, 40, 46, 52, 53, 58
Bioceramics 74
Biohybrid vascular grafts 74
Biomimetic 3, 35, 85, 92, 94, 97, 99, 100, 101, 131
Bioresorbable stents 74, 81, 82, 84, 87

C

Cardiac fibroblasts 106, 110, 111, 112, 113, 116, 117
Cardiac ischemia 6
Cardiac reprogramming 106, 107, 110, 111, 112, 113, 117, 118
Cardiac regeneration 3, 74, 79, 81, 87, 95, 96, 97, 100, 106, 107, 109, 112, 114, 115, 116, 118, 125, 132, 136, 137, 138, 144, 145, 147
Cardiomyocytes 1, 3, 13, 44, 45, 65, 74, 81, 83, 92, 94, 97, 106, 107, 108, 109, 111, 112, 113, 115, 116, 117, 129, 130, 132, 134, 135, 136, 144, 145, 149, 151, 152, 154

D

Dendrimers 17, 33, 40
Drug delivery 13, 22, 43, 47, 52, 61, 77, 79, 95, 96, 100, 126, 131

E

Electrospinning 92, 94, 99, 101, 132

H

Hydrogels 74, 78, 81, 82, 83, 87, 96, 97, 100, 115, 117, 127, 134, 135, 149, 152, 153

I

Implants 74, 77, 78

L

Liposomes 2, 17, 19, 20, 21, 33, 34, 40, 43, 44, 45, 46, 56, 101, 132

M

Mesenchymal stem cells 144
Micelles 12, 17, 19, 22, 34, 42, 46, 57
Microbubble 30, 31, 32, 151, 152

N

Nanocarrier 17, 23, 30, 40, 41, 42, 47, 52, 53, 55, 61, 107
Nanofibers 92, 94, 96, 97, 100, 113, 114, 133, 153
Nanolithography 92, 101
Nanomaterials 1, 2, 8, 21, 101, 106, 117, 118, 125, 127, 131, 133, 154
Nanomedicine 1, 2, 3, 4, 6, 7, 8, 10, 11, 14, 15, 17, 34, 40, 42, 43, 61, 62, 117, 151
Nanoparticles 7, 8, 9, 10, 11, 12, 19, 21, 22, 23, 24, 30, 31, 32, 33, 34, 35, 36, 40, 41, 42, 43, 45, 46, 52, 53, 54, 55, 356, 58, 61, 62, 64, 65, 66, 94, 96, 101, 113, 114,

www.ingramcontent.com/pod-product-compliance
Lightning Source LLC
Chambersburg PA
CBHW041707210326
41598CB00007B/558